INTERMITTENT FASTING *101*

The Complete Guide to Fasting
for Women and Men Over 50.
Heal Your Body Through the
Self-Cleansing Process of Autophagy

ALICIA LYNN

Table of Contents

INTRODUCTION

Within the past few years, the concept of Intermittent Fasting has started to trend heavily, impacting anyone interested in dieting and healthy living. Its origins, however, are much more ancient than most of us would ever think. In this chapter, you'll be introduced to the long history of Intermittent Fasting so that you can better understand how that trajectory leads to today. By the end of this section, you should feel confident that you know where the tradition came from, as well as what it has to do with you—reading this book in this very moment.

IF for Primitive Humans

Intermittent Fasting has been a practice as long as humans have existed. In the times of our most primitive ancestors, IF wasn't so much a chosen lifestyle, as it was a necessity. It came down to the prevalence and availability of food—and the hunter and gatherer's abilities to acquire it.

In these ancient times, people would have had to go longer between meals, and sometimes perhaps spend days without eating. However, what arose from necessity produced incredible and even sustainable physical, mental, and emotional effects. These ancient people would have also (likely unintentionally) been able to concentrate better, live longer, slowing age and digest with ease consistently.

Primitive humans would also occasionally fast for shared purposes once societies and civilizations started assembling. For instance, before going off to war, communities would fast, and young people coming-of-age would fast as part of those rituals. Sometimes societies would also demand a fast as an offering to the gods, or to implore the end of natural disasters such as floods or famines.

Religious Instances of IF

On the same vein as using a fast as an offering to the gods, many ancient cultures eventually required some fasting for their religion purposes. Consider Christianity. Orthodox Christians of the Greek variety still practice their ancient fasts, which comprise almost 200 days out of the year. Non-Orthodox Christians are also invited to fast whenever moved to do so to become closer to the Holy Trinity.

Consider Buddhism. The practice of intermittent fasting has always been essential to reaching enlightenment, because it helps the soul undo its ropes to the body. The enlightened one, Siddhartha, practiced fasting for many years as a method to acquire wisdom.

Consider Judaism. The day before Passover; it is an ancient tradition followed till today that the first-born child of each family should fast to celebrate the miracle from Moses' time that spared all Hebrew first-borns. Furthermore, Jewish people are invited to fast throughout the year at any point to celebrate a life lost, to appeal to God or a prophet, or to express sorrow for a sin or wrong committed.

Consider Islam. The holy month of Ramadan features a 4-week-long fast from the time the sun rises to the time the sun sets. During this time, drinks are also shunned, as well as alcohol drinking, smoking, or performing any bad habits or repetitive practices that don't serve the soul. Muhammad, the prophet of Islam, also suggested that his followers fast every Monday and Thursday (essentially the 5:2 method), but it's unclear how consistently this suggestion is heeded.

Other religions across the world have also required a temporary fast for spiritual reasons, and it is true that many have gotten closer to their gods through this practice. However, there are so many more benefits to fasting than just these spiritual ones, and these other applications are made clear in the next chapters.

From the Past to Now

On top of being used for survival and religious purposes, intermittent fasting has gained appeal through time for its medical applications as well. Even millennia before its trending popularity today, back in 400 BC, intermittent fasting made an appearance and gained popularity by the suggestion of Hippocrates.

Yes, **that** Hippocrates! The infamous "father of modern medicine" advocated for fasting to heal almost any internal injury or state of disease. He once wrote, "To eat when you are sick, is to feed your illness," if that gives you any indication of the incredible uses he found for the practice.

Other ancient Greek philosophers, writers, and historians have echoed these concepts from Hippocrates through time into the early years, AD. Essentially, just like how animals seem to "fast" when they're getting sick or feeling unwell, humans have the same instincts but often ignore them, pushing through the illness and feeding it with food when the body needs the exact opposite.

Past the ancient Greeks, however, other thinkers across time have affirmed the same feelings. For example, Paracelsus (another founder of modern medicine) famously wrote, "Fasting is the greatest remedy," and Benjamin Franklin (one of America's founding fathers) also once inscribed in a journal, "The best of all medicines is resting and fasting."

In the past, fasting has also been used as a form of political protest, and the most famous instance of this happening occurred with Mahatma Gandhi, who lasted 21 days at his longest period of fasting. His goals were to protest against India's dependence on Britain and to acquire freedom and integrity for his people. Many others have taken up fasting for similar aims, but none have been so successful or so famous, it seems.

Contemporary Applications

Now, it seems that fasting has gained new fame in the form of Intermittent Fasting, and the capital letters here are used intentionally to connote the almost "patented" application of these ancient theories in relation to health and weight loss in recent times.

This practice of Intermittent Fasting has been trending for the past few years, and its impact has spread widely since then. People have lost incredible amounts of weight. They've seen their energy levels improve drastically. They've been able to heal brain disorders and reverse the signs of aging. People across the world have come to understand what amazing uses fasting can have, and they are becoming healthier because of these realizations.

Doctors who have practiced fasting cures for decades have almost consistently welcomed the increased interest in IF these days, for they know how much good this practice can do for so many. Fasting is still used for religious and spiritual purposes, and some still practice it as they strive to survive. For others, IF today is revered as the so-called "fountain of youth," and many dietary plans are starting to incorporate its themes.

Overall, it seems that IF has been used throughout time for three main things: survival, spiritual connection, and body/mind health. These applications are valid today, but the focus tends toward that final point in the list: body/mind health. For those seeking a state of internal balance, IF can be a blessing. For those intrigued by IF, keep reading to find out more and to learn how to build this practice into your daily routine.

PART I

NEW MIND, NEW BODY

CHAPTER 1: OVERWEIGHT

Overweight Phenomenon

Intermittent fasting provides numerous benefits to those who are obese, overweight, or have average weight. However, it is not appropriate for everyone, including pregnant and breastfeeding women, as well as those who are dealing with eating disorders and certain health issues.

This is the main reason why you have to study the effects of fasting to you as soon as you begin doing it. Listen to your own body. If you notice some unwanted side effects, find out if it is because your body is just adjusting to the routine or due to more serious issues. If you are extremely worried about the negative side effects, do not hesitate to consult your doctor to ensure your safety.

What Is Obesity?

When your body carries more fat than is defined as healthy for your age and sex, you are said to meet the criteria for obesity. In simple terms, obesity occurs when there is an abnormal or excess amount of body fat, which is known as adipose tissue.

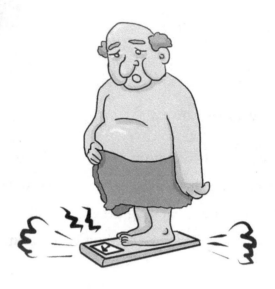

A fat cell is an endocrine cell (a hormone-producing part of your body), and adipose tissue is an endocrine organ. Detailed scientific research has demonstrated that this extra fat in the body produces several "bad chemicals," known as metabolites or cytokines, which have negative influences on health and that ultimately lead to multiple medical problems. Fat produces inflammation (i.e., a fundamental way in which your body reacts to infection, irritation, or any other form of injury), which reinforces the fact that this extra adipose tissue in the body causes various disease processes. Excessive fat can eventually lead to your body becoming resistant to a hormone called insulin, which tries to keep your blood sugar (glucose) in a normal range and ultimately paves the way for development of type 2 diabetes. How Common Is Obesity?

Obesity is one of the most universal chronic diseases. However, there is a pressing need for new guidelines for its medical prevention and treatment.

Do I Weigh Too Much?

You can calculate whether you meet the criteria for overweight or obesity by using a simple mathematical formula involving height and weight; it is called the Body Mass Index (BMI). The numbers derived from this calculation will help you to categorize your weight, as described in just a moment.

It is important to remember that this number can be misleading; it can place some people (e.g., those who are very muscular or who are pregnant or lactating) in a category that does not accurately reflect their disease state.

If your BMI falls between 18.5 and 24.9, you are considered to have a normal weight. However, if your BMI is equal to or greater than 30, you have obesity (Duerenberg et al, 1991).

BMI is the most commonly used tool to assess someone's weight status, and this is what your doctor will commonly use, as well. However, other indicators of excess fat tissue, such as waist circumference, waist-to-hip ratio, and other measures are also used. Waist circumference is used to determine the fat content around your waistline. An excess of abdominal fat or "belly fat" is considered a predictor of risk factors, such as a predisposition to heart disease and type 2 diabetes.

Now, let's talk about how to measure your waist circumference. First, remove any clothing from your waistline.

Stand with your feet shoulders' width apart, and make sure to keep your back straight.

Take two normal breaths, and as you exhale the second breath, tighten the tape measure so that it is snug, but not digging into the skin.

Take the measure of your waist.

Now, all of these steps might seem very complicated. A very easy and accurate way to measure waist circumference is to take the measurement at the belly button or navel. This location often captures the widest circumference, and it is directly related to your risk of metabolic diseases, such as type 2 diabetes and heart disease.

Why Do I Continue to Gain Weight?

Your body sets its own target, or set point, for fat (Schwartz et al, 2000). Fat is our body's fuel supply, the body's gas tank. There are complex signals and mechanisms that regulate the amount of fat in your "tank." Unfortunately, we do not have complete control of the amount of fat in our tank, and there is a common belief in our society that we are able to voluntarily control the balance of fat.

Why Do I Have Trouble Losing Weight?

Many people still believe that obesity is caused simply by eating too many calories and exercising too little. Unfortunately, that's a mistaken belief. How the body regulates weight is similar to how it regulates your water balance. If you need water, your brain makes you thirsty, and you drink. If you drink more than you need, your body gets rid of the excess water. It's the same with calories and body fat. You can control it for a short time by eating less, and you might lose weight.

Can I Lose Weight?

The first step in weight loss is identifying the key contributing factors that are involved in causing obesity, which varies from person to person. There is not a "one size fits all" approach. The reason behind this is that there are many types of obesity and, as a result, it is necessary to try multiple therapies and combinations of therapies to help different people achieve a healthy weight. Dietary changes might work well for one person, whereas another person might lose weight by improving their sleep habits. We should not expect that there's a simple solution for how you can achieve and maintain a healthy weight. It is critical to understand that obesity is caused by varied biological and physiological disruptions in different people, and it is important to match every person to their ideal weight with an individualized treatment approach, through exposure to several different methods. Through this strategy, you are most likely to achieve beneficial results and to lose weight. Although interventions (such as engaging in consistent exercise, eating a high-quality diet, practicing stress reduction, and developing good sleep patterns) are at the cornerstone of efforts to achieve and maintain a healthy weight, other individuals might need more invasive interventions (such as medical and surgical interventions) to achieve weight loss. There are multiple medical options available for the treatment of obesity (Apovian et al, 2015). You should talk to your doctor about an appropriate referral to a practitioner trained in obesity medicine, who will complete an interview and a physical examination to decide on the best line of treatment for you. In conclusion, because obesity is a complex disease, it often needs multiple methods to achieve the desired result of weight loss.

Can Obesity Be Prevented?

Considering the current obesity epidemic, policy makers and national agencies are evaluating various methods and designing programs to help build an environment that can support a healthy lifestyle and ultimately prevent obesity. However, considering the complex and multidimensional etiologies of obesity, it remains a public-health problem.

How Does My Body Process and Store Fat?

Regulation of body weight and fat tissue appears to be coordinated primarily by our brains. A small area within our brain called the hypothalamus receives information from a variety of sources in our body. A hormone, called leptin, provides information to the brain about the body's energy stores (Friedman and Halaas, 1998). Signals also reach the brain from other organs of your body, such as the pancreas and the liver, which give information about the energy demands and nutrients availability for the resting energy expenditure, and communicates this information to the brain. In terms of food intake, signals about the type, smell, taste, and texture of food are sent to the higher brain centers; these signals along with the others from various organs direct you to start or to stop eating. Overall, the hypothalamus integrates and orchestrates this mass of information and works to achieve a fat set point, which it views as normal for one's body. The storage of fat happens in alignment with this principle, with a constant need to maintain and to achieve that physiological set point.

Where on My Body Is Fat Likely to Develop?

There are different kinds of fat in our body: brown, white, subcutaneous (mostly concentrated in your hips, butt, and thighs), and visceral (mostly in your mid-section). Depending on your gender, race, age, and ethnicity, you might have a predisposition to accumulate different kinds of fat in various parts of your body. For example, women tend to accumulate more fat around their hips and thighs, whereas men are likely to accumulate it around their bellies (so-called abdominal fat). Abdominal fat conveys a greater health risk than does hip or thigh fat. This translates to a greater impact on insulin resistance, which increases the risk of diabetes, increases your total cholesterol levels, and predisposes you to an increased risk of stroke and heart disease (Schneider et al, 2010).

How Does Being Overweight Jeopardize My Health and Well-Being?

Obesity is now known to have caused or exacerbated more than 40 distinct disorders that lead to poor health and an overall decreased quality of life (Cummings et al, 2002). The medical complications (or co-morbidities) range from metabolic problems (such as type 2 diabetes mellitus, high cholesterol levels), to high blood pressure, gallstones, fatty liver disease, pancreatitis, obstructive sleep apnea, and even reproductive dysfunction. Other diseases that are often associated with obesity include stress incontinence (an inability to control your urination), increased pressure within your brain (idiopathic intracranial hypertension), which leads to headaches, degenerative joint disease (also known as arthritis), and vertebral disc disease. Scientific research has also provided evidence of a strong association between obesity and many cancers.

Is Obesity Inherited?

So far, we have learned that obesity is a complex condition that results from multiple interactions with hereditary and environmental factors. It is now well established that different forms of obesity tend to concentrate within families. Obesity risk is two to eight times greater for someone with a family history, as opposed to a person with no family history of obesity; there is an even higher risk observed in those with severe obesity (Zlot et al, 2007).

Studies on twins have compared those who were raised together to those who were raised in a different environment; these investigators have affirmed that genetic influences on BMI are substantial (Stunkard et al, 1990).

There are other rare causes of genetic obesity in which a single gene is affected and leads to more severe forms of obesity; these forms of obesity are seen most often in early childhood. In summary, in most cases, genetic variation influences a person's predisposition for developing obesity, but environmental and psychological factors contribute significantly to the manifestation. Our understanding of how genes that contribute to weight and to energy regulation continues to advance rapidly.

Am I More Likely to Gain Weight as I Age?

Aging is characterized by changes in body composition. Imaging studies demonstrate that as we age, subcutaneous fat (the fat below the skin) decreases and the visceral fat (fat in the abdominal region) increases. Visceral fat is not a good thing to have, as we have discussed previously. It is associated with systemic inflammation, and it continues to increase the risk for coronary artery disease, stroke, and death. Another important age-related change along with altered body composition is loss of muscle mass. Muscle helps us maintain a high metabolic rate and an increased resting energy expenditure. Therefore, its loss is associated with a reduction in the total energy expenditure.

The altered body composition and loss of muscle mass leads to fat gain.

Both increases in visceral fat and decreases in muscle mass are linked to a loss of sensitivity to insulin. The lower the sensitivity to insulin, the more the body secretes insulin. This metabolic hormone causes a torrent of problems, given that it's a storage hormone. It helps to increase the uptake of glucose and fat production while decreasing the burning of fat and stored glucose (glycogen).

What Can I Do About My Excess Weight?

There are multiple effective treatment options available to lose weight. To decide which type of treatment will be best suited for your needs, you will need a comprehensive evaluation, completed by a physician trained in obesity medicine. In addition, consultation with a nutritionist as well as a psychologist is also of vital importance. After you have obtained a thorough evaluation, which can include blood testing, your doctor and the entire team will decide on a management plan with you.

The various treatment options available include behavioral, medical, and surgical options. Behavioral treatment involves making lifestyle modifications (such as making better food choices, incorporating more hours of exercise in your routine, and maintaining a healthy and consistent sleep schedule).

If your doctor thinks that making lifestyle modifications will not be helpful by themselves (which is often related to a history of consistent lifestyle changes, severe obesity, or moderate obesity with many obesity co-morbidities (e.g., high blood pressure, type 2 diabetes, obstructive sleep apnea), he or she might choose to prescribe a medicine. There are various weight-loss medicines available that might be used to lose weight; however, only a doctor may prescribe these for you. After you start on a medication, you need to be followed to assess the benefits and side effects of the medicine. These medications are prescribed for long-term use, as discontinuing these medications often leads to weight gain.

CHAPTER 2: WHAT IS EMOTIONAL EATING

What is Emotional eating?

As even non-professionals eventually come to notice, mental and physical illnesses are categorized by various qualifiers among members of the healthcare professions. These qualifiers include "disease" (i.e., Lyme disease), "condition" (i.e., psychological condition), and "syndrome" (i.e., toxic-shock syndrome), but few laymen understand the distinctions. Nonetheless, it is quite important to understand how this categorization pertains to this eating "disorder," as it brings clarification to how science views this illness, and how treatment is meant to affect it.

Despite the many physical aspects associated with BED (physical comorbidities), binge-eating disorder is regarded as a psychological rather than physical ailment (an aberrant social behavior), best managed by psychological therapy. That is not to say that medical doctors and other therapeutic practitioners cannot be helpful in alleviating many of the symptoms associated with binge-eating disorder, only that such approaches treat the symptoms, not the source(s) of the problem. Thus the first step to understanding binge-eating disorder is to acknowledge that you are dealing with a serious psychological issue—that manifests physically.

29

Do you suffer from emotional eating?

Obesity levels amongst people are certainly higher than they have ever been in history. This trend has spread throughout the world. People are gaining weight at excessive rates. But the big question is, why? What is it that is really causing people to gain weight?

The quick answer is to blame it on the junk food, and that would be the logical answer. There are so many food manufacturing companies that are creating junk foods which are not healthy for people to consume.

Junk foods are basically processed foods that have been altered from their natural state. The common junk foods contain added pesticides, preservatives, flavorings, sugars, salts, seasonings and all kinds of things that are bad for our health.

Unnatural foods will cause you to feel unnatural. In other words, they will cause you to feel symptoms of stress, anxiety, irritation, irregular heart beat and more.

Even though these symptoms may be natural in some life circumstances, when they are caused simply by food, then they are unnatural.

The Real Reason

We know junk food is the problem for the majority of health problems in America and other developed countries. Until government agencies ban junk foods from being sold in the supermarkets, they are always going to be there and people will always buy them.

It is no surprise to ordinary citizens that junk food is bad for them when they see it in the supermarkets. They know cookies, cakes, pizza, and fried foods are just going to make them feel lousy after they eat them. But they continue to eat these foods anyway. So again, why?

The real reason has to do with stress more than anything else. People live such stressful lives in the modern age. They have to worry about making a living, taking care of their kids, and so on. It gets to a point where they really have no time to relax and feel comfortable at all.

People in stressful situations tend to form bad habits in order to relieve their stress. One of the biggest habits people develop is binge eating on junk food.

Once this happens, the unnatural chemicals and additives in those foods will raise their stress levels even higher. Therefore, instead of treating the problem, junk food just makes it worse.

The Stress Factor on Weight Gain

Stress, if not checked, becomes a significant factor in weight gain because it leads to emotional eating. For example, most people, in an attempt to battle with stress, especially at work, find themselves eating a tub of ice cream, emotionally and mindlessly. Others, in an effort to beat tight work deadlines, furiously eat fries and hamburgers in front of their computers. Maybe you are a busy mom, and you have to drop the kids to school before rushing to work and engage yourself in moving back and forth to meet tight deadlines for various appointments and a series of meetings. Before you know it, you find yourself with no time to eat mindfully, and you emotionally begin to over-eat cookies in your car. Perhaps you are desperately trying to make things work as a small business owner, only to wake up one day and notice that there is a considerable expansion on your waistline. If you find yourself incarcerated in any of these scenarios, you are not alone, and chances remain high that it is not your fault. Such stress creates a fertile ground for weight gain, especially when it goes on for a long time. First, it makes it hard for us to implement a healthy lifestyle due to the interference it has on our willpower to so do. Second, it enhances our appetite for emotional eating and makes hold onto the fat, which begins to accumulate in our bodies.

Therefore, what are the biology and psychology behind overeating and weight gain related to stress? Let us look at some of the reasons that make stress a factor in weight gain.

Stress and Hormones

A release of a cascade of hormones such as cortisol, adrenaline, and CRH is triggered in the body in the event where the brain detects any form of danger or threat. Whether you are facing your harsh boss, battling to pay a big credit card bill, or rushing from place to place to meet tight deadlines, the brain signals your body to release these chemicals to help deal with the threat. These hormones are meant to prepare your body and the brain to tackle the danger by making you ready to withstand it, or alert to take action.

In preparation for fight-or-fright, adrenaline makes the blood to rush into your muscles in the short-term, flowing from the internal organs; hence making you less angry. However, the stress hormone, which is known as cortisol, lingers long after the effects of adrenaline have worn off. This hormone begins to signal the body for more food supply. Remember, your neuroendocrine system does not get the difference in the kind of a threat you are facing. Our ancestors required a lot of energy to battle with wild animals, so they needed more storage of glucose and fat in their bodies.

However, today, we sit before our computers working for long hours to meet tight deadlines or relax on our coaches worrying about how to settle bills at the end of the month. Unlike our ancestors who worked with much energy, dealing with the kind of threats and dangers they faced, the type of stressors we face today do not work with much energy form our bodies. Nevertheless, the mind cannot capture the difference, because there is no such an update in our neuroendocrine system. Therefore, you find yourself reaching for an extra plate of cookies, hamburger, or fries to replenish your body's food supply. The brain treats any form of stress as a threat and attempts to prepare your body to deal with it. You find yourself overeating, and consequently gaining more weight.

Stress and Belly Fat

Belly fat and weight gain around our middles have been directly linked to chronic stress. Many people live in fear of the unknown. The problem is that the body cannot make the difference between life-threatening anxiety and stress that comes as a result of work pressures. Being late to capture the train, or anxiety that occurs as a result of battling to settle debts and pay bills is treated the same as having to run away from a collapsing building. All these stressors are treated the same, and the brain takes the initiative to release adrenaline and cortisol to prepare us for flight or fight, just as it did to our ancestors when they battled life-threatening tigers and lions.

Nowadays, the kind of stress we face does not require us to fight or flee as a result of modern lifestyle, and it happens to be continuous. Therefore, after going through stressful moments either at work or in your relationship, cortisol levels are going to remain high, and your appetite for food will increase. Your body still thinks that you need to refuel your energy stores for glucose and fat after battling such a stressor through fighting and fleeing. That is why when you are leading a stressful life, you constantly feel hungry. You end up craving carbohydrates and fats because there is a bodily urge to stock up on energy foods. Therefore, when you are under chronic stress, your body expects that you should fight or run to flee a threat or danger. If you do not, the body ends up depositing the glucose and the fat in your system as belly fat around your middle. Such fat deposits target the belly because it is close to the liver, and if energy is required, it can be quickly reached out and converted as needed. Cortisol –the stress hormone – slows down the body's metabolism in an attempt to help the body sustain enough glucose supply for the hard physical and mental work of combating your stressors. You end up burning less fat than you should, leading to more accumulation of the belly fat, hence abdominal weight gain.

Stress and Anxiety

During the fight/ flight response, which is activated by adrenaline in the event of a threat or danger, we tend to get active and fidgety. Anxiety kicks in, and you feel wired-up as adrenaline responds to the threat of stress. You find that you feel unsettled, and you may begin to run around anxiously, reaching out for a solution. Such anxiety triggers emotional eating. In an attempt to calm down, you find yourself eating or overeating unhealthy foods. This is a prevalent response to stress.

Anxiety makes you eat mindlessly, and you find yourself eating more without getting satisfied. You cannot even tell how much you have eaten because you are busy churning worrisome and stressful thoughts around your head, to the point where you cannot even focus on the taste of your food. You eat more emotionally and less mindfully, when you are anxious and stressed, and you feel less satisfied, however more you may eat. This emotional and anxious overeating leads to weight gain.

Stressful Cravings and fast food

Chronic stress comes with the tendency to crave foods that give us short-term comforts, such as ice creams, hamburgers, freshly baked cookies, and potato chips. These foods are highly processed and easy to eat, with high levels of salt, sugar, or fat.

Such craving has both psychological and biological reasons. We may end up craving more sugar and fat as a result of our brain's reward system being messed up by both stress and high cortisol level in the body. In addition, we tend to reach out for childhood memories during such stressful moments that associate comfort with such sweet foods.

Since it takes mental energy and time to plan and cook a well-balanced meal, you find yourself unable to do it. More likely, you drive to the fast-food joint to reward yourself with these highly processed foods. Most people who live and work in urban areas are less likely to cook and eat dinner at home because of traffic jams, which lead to increased stress as you commute from work to your house. You get home late; feeling hungrier with your willpower substantially interfered with.

The only option you have is to drive to the nearby food joint and get something for supper. You find yourself eating unhealthy foods mindlessly and emotionally, which leads to weight gain due to high levels of salt, fat, and sugar in such foods.

Less Sleep

More than 40% of Americans lie awake at night due to stress, according to APA's survey, which focused on Stress in America. At night, you may find yourself lying awake at night, worrying about how you will pay your bills, your work-related issues, and relationship issues. You worry about who will look after your kids when you leave home for work. Research links worry about being a significant insomnia cause. The mind refuses to switch off, as a result of being overactive. If you are a student, you may find yourself spending sleepless nights to write notes or cram for your exams. At such times, you may lose sleep because your mind and body are under intense stress due to such a last-minute rush.

Such stress results in fatigue due to decreased levels of blood sugar. You even end up disrupting your sleep cycle further if you force yourself to stay awake by drinking caffeinated drinks or coffee. Other people resort to drinking alcohol to feel better during such stressful moments making the situation worse off.

When it comes to influencing weight loss or weight gain, sleep is a significant factor. Leptin and ghrelin are the hormones that regulate appetite, and their functioning may be disrupted by lack of sleep. You will tend to crave foods with high levels of sugars such as carbs when you are grumpy or tired as a result of lacking enough sleep. Your will power will also get eroded by lack of sleep, and you will easily fall for the temptations to eat unhealthy foods mindlessly and emotionally. This will lead to weight gain as a result of sleep deprivation.

Stress-induced eating habits

Many people experience changes in their eating behaviors when under high levels of stress. Let us quickly look at some of these dietary changes, and how they lead to weight gain. Here is a quick summary:

High-fat and high-sugar food consumption – these foods are unhealthy and tend to result in weight gain. Mainly, they are processed foods that are sugary, salty, and fatty. Unfortunately, people tend to crave these processed foods while experiencing chronic stress, hence gaining more weight.

Eating emotionally - due to excess nervous energy, anxiety, and increased level of cortisol, you find yourself craving unhealthy foods and eating more food than you usually eat. When you reach for a second helping or engage yourself in emotional snacking, you tend to get some temporary stress relief. Before you know it, you find yourself accumulating more fat and gaining weight.

Eating more fast foods –you forgo cooking a well-balanced, healthy dinner at home and you find yourself eating fast foods which have high levels of fat and sugar. You are also likely to emotionally and mindlessly eat larger portion sizes due to chronic stress.

Too busy to exercise – remember that one of the reasons most people live under chronic stress is because they have hectic schedules. That means exercise is the last thing they can think of, and it becomes non-existence in their to-do list. Long working hours, commuting stress and staring at the TV when one gets home, leaves no time for exercise. This leads to more weight gain. Forgetting to drink water – you end up confusing being thirsty with being hungry in a busy schedule, trying to deal with various life challenges. The net result is that you eat more, while hardly drinking enough water, hence gaining more weight due to overeating.

Skipping meals –you skip taking your breakfast to avoid getting late for work or fail to eat your lunch because your to-do list has many things demanding for your attention. Eating a healthy meal is no longer a priority because you are struggling to juggle a dozen things in your busy schedule. Such stress makes you to emotionally and mindlessly overeat, because you are not sure whether you will get little time to eat again.

Trying fad diets - when you realize that you are gaining weight, you get into another cycle of stress. You find yourself trying harmful fad diets or eating less food than your body requires in an attempt to shed down the excess weight. You forget taking a balanced meal of carbohydrates, proteins, vegetables, and fruits.

Such dangerous diets may be attractive in the short run, but they tend to be harmful to your health in the long run. They lead to emotional and mindless eating, which results in more weight gain.

Sleep deprivation – when stressed up, many tend to remain awake at night, worrying about their busy schedules, relationships, and their kids. Their will power is eroded, and the rate of metabolism slows down due to lack of sleep. The results in forgetting to eat mindfully, hence resorting to emotional eating habits, which lead to weight gain.

Breaking the stress and weight gain cycle

It is not easy to break the cycle of stress and weight gain. This is because when you realize that you have gained more weight and your clothes no longer fit well, that by itself can fuel your stress cycle. Remember that the more stressed you are, the more susceptible you are to gain weight. It will take willpower to break this cycle. That notwithstanding, you can combat stress and weight changes that come about with it, by taking some concrete steps.

Make exercise a priority – when it comes to busting stress and shed off unwelcome weight gain, exercise is a crucial component that you need to integrate into your schedule. Simultaneously, exercise can knock down stress, while warding off any weight gain related to it. Remain physically active after work, by either jogging around the neighborhood, going to the gym, or taking an evening walk. Aerobic activities will be the best to help you deal with stress-related weight gain.

Mind your eating habits – being mindful of what you eat is essential to help you regulate and gain control of your food consumption habits. Stop eating emotionally and mindlessly by keeping a journal of what you eat. You need a food diary, or an app to monitor your eating habits. You will be able to improve your eating habits by being mindful of every food that you put in your mouth. Have an eating program and prepare well-balanced meals for yourself at home.

Find other rewarding activities unrelated to food – you are less likely to overeat when you have other activities to act as a stress buster. However hectic your schedule might be, you need to set aside some time to unwind and relieve yourself of any form of stress so that you can improve your mood, refresh your mind, and think more clearly. You can go for a massage, make time for being with friends and family members, pat your dog, read a book, take a hike or go for a yoga class. Such activities will help you ward off any weight gain related to stress and cut the cycle of stress, which comes as a result of busy schedules or any other stressor in your life.

CHAPTER 3: NO DIET, BUT NEW LIFE!

Intermittent fasting changes your lifestyle to a certain degree. You learn to say "no" during certain hours and friends will be supportive of you when they know that you are serious. During the hours of fasting, you need to make sure that you get sufficient rest. People underestimate the power of sleep. During the hours of sleep, you are burning off calories, and your body is also put into repair mode. Thus, because you are feeding your body less, you need to take your sleep hours very seriously. Make sure that you get at least eight hours of good quality sleep because this helps you to get through the hours of fasting and to feel refreshed in the morning.

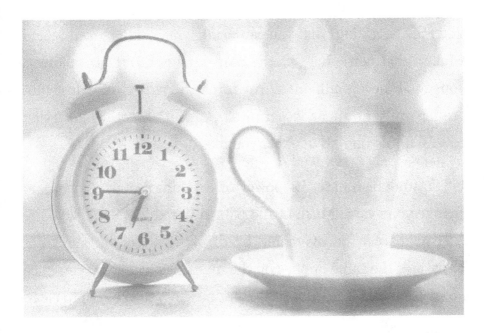

A certain amount of exercise is beneficial while you are fasting. As this is a fast to lose weight and shape up, the best time for any strenuous type of exercise could be before the evening meal or before lunch as well, if it fits with your lifestyle. If you don't like exercise very much, there are several exercises you can do that are fun rather than seen as a chore. For example, a DVD of Zumba-style dance is a great encouragement to get up on your feet and dance in a way that exercises the different parts of the body. It's fun, and therefore you don't see it as exercise. Similarly, taking the dog out for a walk was a good way of getting exercise that is good for the heart health. Walking will always be useful since it gets all of your body parts ticking over in a very healthy way.

You may be asking what you can drink while you are fasting and I found that nettle tea was the best thing of all. It tastes sweet; you don't need milk in it. An infusion or tea that does not require milk or sugar is permitted, and it's worthwhile trying several until you find one that you like.

If you underestimate the power of drinking water, it's time to change your view. Much of the pain suffered by people who are overweight can be overcome by drinking water on a regular basis, and the same applies on the mornings when you can have little else for your breakfast. Water does help the system to clean out, and it also has another role. It feeds your muscles and stops them from cramping up through dehydration. In my teaching of intermittent fasting, I am always surprised by people who dismiss dehydration as a cause of their pain. They see this as being something drastic that only happens to hospital patients. Unfortunately, if you don't drink sufficient water, it is going on inside you, whether you admit it or not. Your body needs water and on a regular basis.

Something that I also encourage people to try while fasting is meditation. This helps them to relax and makes them much more aware of the changes that are going on within the body. Fasting becomes something that isn't hard. It is seen as giving back, and those who meditate can stay calm and focused on their diet that is always useful. They are also less likely to cheat. The calmness that you can derive from meditation makes the whole process much easier, especially if you opt to fast for 24 hours at a time. The energy you would typically obtain from food can be gained from meditation, and that's somewhat important when you are fasting for such a long period.

It's important that you prepare for your diet and that you are mentally capable of getting through the fasting period without feeling too anxious about needing to eat. In the first couple of days, you may have minor pangs of hunger, but since you know that you will be eating soon, this is usually something that is easy to overcome. Meditation may help you, if you find the last few hours of a fast difficult to cope with.

What to Expect When starting your new journey of life

Setting your expectations before committing to a fast is an excellent way of preparing both your body and mind for the lifestyle and dietary changes that are about to happen.

Before delving into the details of these expectations, you should be clear first about your personal objectives for the fast. Here are some common scenarios that have led people into fasting:

They want to lose weight, and gain a leaner body.

They have tried other popular diets before, and they felt dissatisfied with the process or frustrated over the results.

They want to significantly improve the current condition of their body.

They want to live a longer, healthier, and more productive life.

Fasting is a proven method of losing weight in a healthy manner, while also increasing your energy levels. For many, it is a life-changing practice that has enabled them to achieve their other personal goals in life.

Committing to a fast requires determination and confidence that you can go through this without giving in to your old ways. You need plan to prepare for this because you might have to make drastic changes in your life.

For your guidance, here are the various things that you should expect when starting a fast:

Grocery Shopping

Fasting would significantly change the way you shop for food. Aside from the frequency of your shopping days, some items from your current shopping list must be removed and replaced with healthier alternatives.

In general, you should stick to leaner types of proteins, such as certain types of fishes and egg whites. For fruits and vegetables, it is advisable to spend a bit more and buy organic produce.

Meal Restrictions

The exact meal schedule that you have to observe depends on the fasting method that you are following. However, all fasting methods would limit your calorie intake either by reducing the allowable number of calories, or by urging you to skip certain meals—if not all of them.

For example, a 5:2 diet imposes a 500-calorie limit among women, and 600-calorie limit among men. Both are significantly less than the recommended amount for average individuals.

Imbibing alcohol drinks during a fast is strongly discouraged as well. Even when you are on your "off days" from your fast, experts recommend only a moderate amount.

During a fast, you would also have to drink more water. If you prefer flavored beverages, then you should stick to herbal teas and black coffee with no sugar. Some health experts also allow drinking club soda during a fast.

Refer to chapter 4 of this book for more information about the meal restrictions of different fasting methods.

Physiological side-effects

Many of these side-effects can be considered as the disadvantages of fasting. However, with the right mindset, you would be able to power through them despite the challenges they might pose to your day-to-day life.

Your body will enter its fasting state at around 8 hours after your last meal. This is the average duration for a full digestion and complete absorption of nutrients from the food and beverages you have consumed prior to your fasting period.

It could vary, however, depending on the kind of meal you had—for instance, foods high in fiber need a longer digestive period compared to leafy vegetables.

During the initial fasting period, your body would still get most of its energy from your glucose or glycogen stores.

The glycogen stored in your liver would be depleted after an overnight fast.

Once your body has completely used up all the glucose stores in your body, it would begin sourcing energy from the fat stores within your body.

Take note, however, that the body is already converting fat into energy even before you have consumed all the glycogen in your body. Fasting only increases the rate of fat-burning, thus making it an effective means of losing excess weight.

There's no right fasting scheme. The essential thing is to choose one that works best for you. Some people get results with shorter fasts; others may require longer fasts. Some people make classic water-just fast; others make tea and coffee quickly, others a bone broth. Regardless of what you do, keeping hydrated, and monitoring yourself is very important. You should stop immediately if you feel ill at any point. You might be hungry, but don't feel sick.

Knowing what to expect is critical in the long-term success of your fast. Realign your goals based on what you have learned from this chapter so that you can create a realistic and achievable fasting plan.

PART II

NEW BODY, NEW LIFE

CHAPTER 4: WHAT IS AUTOPHAGY?

The word autophagy means something eating itself, and that is exactly what triggers the reduction of body mass in humans. Your body stays in the growth mode when you eat regularly. It generates energy to do work by using food molecules. The cells store the extra energy inside them in the form of fat. The waste products that enter the cells in the body (due to internal and external factors) gather inside them. This affects your organs, tissues, and eventually, your health and weight too.

However, when you stop eating and start fasting, your body starts looking for sources of energy. As a result, the fat stored in the cells is broken down, and energy is released from them. Therefore, autophagy is a process where the body cells destroy their damaged parts and proteins and then recycle them in order to build themselves.

You can also view autophagy as a process where the cells in the body burn away the toxins stored in them and then use the remains to make something new. Many tissues and organs start the process of autophagy when they are deprived of food.

But How Does Your Body Know When To Start The Process Of Autophagy?

A signal must be sent to the organs to start breaking down the cells to produce energy. This can be done in many ways. It is not just fasting that can start autophagy in your body. Here are some other ways of losing weight that you can opt for.

Exercise

The more stress you create in the muscles and cells of your body, the more strongly the cellular cleanup phase will be triggered. All the extensive forms of exercise, including jogging, sprinting, weight training and physical training, regulate autophagy by inducing stress in the body. When the body is highly worked up, it needs energy that it gains by burning up the cellular waste.

Cold Showers

Yes, cold showers can also invoke healthy autophagy inside you. Studies have shown that people who swim during the winter exhibit higher levels of cell repair and recycling. Therefore, taking cold showers regularly can help you lose weight and stay healthy.

Steam Bath

Subjecting yourself to high temperatures through saunas and steam baths generates heat stress inside you. This heat results in the destruction and recycling of cancerous as well as damaged cells.

A trip to a spa can be good for relaxing, rejuvenating, losing weight and continuously preventing diseases. Besides, exposing yourself to strong heat also helps to cure depression by naturally releasing heat shock proteins.

Intermittent Fasting

There are indicators in your body that activate or cease certain processes. The hormonal levels are one of them. When you begin intermittent fasting, you deprive the cells of essential nutrients. This activates the hormone glucagon in the body. This hormone works in opposition to insulin. While insulin increases blood sugar levels, glucagon brings them down to maintain the balance. The two hormones are like the ends of a see-saw.

When you are fasting, insulin levels go down, and, as a result, glucagon levels go up. This rise triggers autophagy. Your body gets the message that it is time to break down the stored fats in the body cells to increase the insulin levels again.

Antioxidants

Though antioxidants do not directly invoke the process of autophagy in your body, they have been known to indirectly work towards it. Foods rich in antioxidants support the process when you are fasting, which in turn ensures that you undergo a healthy and balanced autophagy process.

Is There Something That Can Stop Autophagy?

There are factors that can stop your autophagy process. The major one is the mTOR. It stops the autophagy in your body when there are enough nutrients in the cells. It is highly sensitive, and eating as little as 50 calories can increase the level of mTOR.

If you consume fats, it might not raise your insulin levels, and it might keep the mTOR levels suppressed. Nevertheless, high amounts of ketones and fats would break your fast.

Here is a list of things that you can take to keep your insulin levels low and let your body continue the waste removal process of your cells:

Green Tea

Coconut Oil

MCT Oil

Ginger compounds

Galangal

Reishi mushroom extracts

Black coffee

Apple cider vinegar

All these items can help to boost autophagy in your body.

Is It Just For Weight Loss?

Absolutely not. When the cells renew themselves by burning up the waste inside them, they do more than decrease your weight. Clean and healthy cells decrease the risk of developing diseases. Many forms of cancer, neurodegenerative diseases like Alzheimer's and Parkinson's, and metabolic and autoimmune diseases can be prevented through autophagy.

It helps fight infectious diseases and regulates inflammation. It has also been associated with fighting depression and schizophrenia. Fasting-induced autophagy is very helpful in keeping you healthy and preventing medical conditions. It is always good to get rid of the waste around and inside you. A clean environment is healthy and keeps you from getting sick.

Here is a list of major benefits of autophagy, both inside and outside of a body cell.

Increases metabolism

Decreases oxidative stress

Increases genomic stability that prevents cancer

Eliminates waste from the body

Increases neuroendocrine homeostasis

Decreases inflammation

Increases lifespan

Eliminates aging cells

Improves muscle performance

Does Autophagy Help Women? How?

The ghrelin or the hunger hormone increases more quickly in women than in men. Women start feeling hungry again quickly after having a meal. Their bodies start craving for food much faster and, therefore, are under more stress to look for energy sources. The cleansing of their body cells makes them immune to catching diseases and helps them to develop a stronger immune system.

Does Autophagy Have Anti-Aging Effects Too?

Consider a real-life example. Assume that you have two cars, X and Y. You are somehow biased towards car X, and so you take much better care of it. You wash it every day, get it serviced every few months, and refuel the tank. On the other hand, car Y does not see many bright days. It is just a backup option for you for the days X is out for servicing or repairs. You do not get its tank refueled, it stays covered in dirt and has been out for just one servicing in years.

Now, which car do you think would last longer? Obviously, car X. When you pay attention to health and get the repairs done on time, faults and damages do not pile up. Your car X would stay as good as new even after years of driving, but car Y would start causing trouble very soon.

The same thing happens with the cells in your body. When the non-functional components and cellular waste keeps sitting inside the cell, it degrades your health and makes you look older. But when they keep recycling and renewing, it shows on your skin. Rejuvenated and youthful cells make your skin softer and healthier.

Autophagy is like a cellular garbage disposal system. Newer cells wash away the dead and unhealthy ones. This leads to increased elimination of aging cells. Autophagy slows down the aging mechanism of your body, which makes you look younger and healthier for a long time.

How Does Your Body Renew Itself Through Autophagy?

Small things matter, and when it comes to aging, small things are the only ones that matter. Cells are what keep you healthy and sick. They store energy, carry oxygen and do everything for your body. In addition, they are the ones that keep you from aging on the inside and outside.

Let us understand how this works. The cells in your body are continuously at work, so they experience a lot of wear and tear. The over-used cells eventually stop working, thus becoming useless. When this happens, the production of new and healthy cells is also discouraged by the useless ones.

These used up cells are known as senescent cells. A senescent cell is a living cell, but its functioning does not contribute to maintaining person's health. And while they do not contribute to anything, they do not let new cells to get formed in the body either. Over the years, the senescent cells keep accumulating in the body. They perform just baseline functions, stop the creation of new cells and promote inflammation. The worst part for women is that they speed up the aging of the nearby cells.

Autophagy clears away the damaged cells, thus making way for the youthful cells to appear. You stay young, healthy and energetic for a long period. Therefore, working towards burning up the waste in your body cells is a great thing for you to do.

Developing healthy habits in your life is a good way to live. No one likes an untidy home, while a shining home with new furniture is loved by all, including the ones who live there. Autophagy is a way to throw away all the old things from home and make space for refreshing new things.

***

Studies on intermittent fasting

What you may be surprised to know is that most of us already fast each day when we are sleeping. You could extend the natural fast time for a little bit longer. For example, you may decide to skip breakfast and have your first meal at noon and your last meal at 8 pm. This would be considered a form of intermittent fasting.

With this method, you technically fast for sixteen hours each day and then only eat during an eight-hour period of the day. This form of fasting, also known as the 16/8 method, is one of the popular options when it comes to intermittent fasting.

Despite what you may be thinking right now, intermittent fasting is actually easier than you think. It doesn't take much planning and countless people who have gone on this diet report that they feel better and have more energy when they are on a fast. In the beginning, you may struggle a bit with hunger, but it won't take long before your body adapts and gets used to it.

Why fast?

The next question that you may have is why you should consider fasting in the first place. Humans have actually been going through periods of fasting for many years. Sometimes they did this because it was a necessity since they were not able to find any food to eat. Then there were also times that the fasting was done for religious reasons. Religions such as Buddhism, Christianity, and Islam mandate some form of fasting. Also, it is natural to fast when you are feeling sick.

Although fasting sometimes has a negative connotation, there is really nothing that is unnatural about fasting. In fact, our bodies are well equipped to handle times when we have to go without eating. There are quite a few processes inside of the body that changes when we go on a fast. This helps our bodies to continue functioning during periods of famine.

When we fast, we get a significant reduction in insulin and blood sugar levels, as well as a drastic increase in what is known as the human growth hormone. While this was something that was originally done when food was scarce, it is now used to help people to lose weight. With fasting, burning fat becomes simple, easier, and effective.

Some people decide to go on a fast because it can help their metabolism. This kind of fasting is good for improving various health disorders and diseases. There is also some evidence that shows how intermittent fasting can help you to live longer. Studies show that rodents were able to extend their lifespan with intermittent fasting.

Other research shows that fasting can help protect against various diseases such as Alzheimer's, cancer, type-2 diabetes, and heart disease. Then, there are those who choose to go on an intermittent fast because it's convenient for their lifestyle. Fasting can be a really effective life hack. For instance, the fewer meals you have to make, the simpler your life will become.

Why does intermittent fasting work?

When you begin intermittent fasting, you will most likely keep your calorie intake the same, but rather than spreading your meals throughout the day, you will eat bigger meals during a shorter time frame. For example, rather than eating 3 to 4 meals a day, you might eat one large meal at 11 am, then another large meal at 6 pm, with no meals in between 11 am and 6 pm, and after 6 pm, no meals until 11 am the next day. This is only one method of intermittent fasting, and others will be detailed in this book in later chapters. However, you first must understand why this method works.

Intermittent fasting is a method utilized by many bodybuilders, athletes, and fitness gurus to keep their muscle mass high and their body fat percentage low. It is a simple strategy that allows you to eat the foods you enjoy, while still promoting fat loss and muscle gain or maintenance. Intermittent fasting can be practiced short term or long term, but the best results come from adopting this method into your daily lifestyle.

Though the word "fasting" may alarm the average person, intermittent fasting does not equate to starving yourself. To understand the principles behind successful intermittent fasting, we'll first go over the body's two states digestion: the fed state and the fasting state.

For three to five hours after eating a meal, your body is in what is known as the "fed state." During the fed state, your insulin levels increase to absorb and digest your food. When your insulin levels are high, it is very difficult for your body to burn fat. Insulin is a hormone produced by the pancreas to regulate glucose levels in the bloodstream. Though its purpose is to regulate, insulin is technically a storage hormone. When insulin levels are high, your body is burning your food for energy, rather than your stored fat, which is why increased levels of it prevent weight loss.

After the three to five hours are up, your body has finished processing the meal, and you enter the post-absorptive state. The post-absorptive state lasts anywhere from 8 to 12 hours. After this time gap, is when your body enters the fasted state. Since your body has completely processed your food by this point, your insulin levels are low, making your stored fat extremely accessible for burning.

In the fasted state, your body has no food left to utilize for energy, so your stored fat is burned instead. Intermittent fasting allows your body to reach an advanced fat burning state that you would normally reach with the average, 'three meals per day' eating pattern. This factor alone is the reason why many people notice rapid results with intermittent fasting without even making changes to their exercise routines, how much they eat, or what they eat. They are simply changing the timing and pattern of their food intake.

When you begin an intermittent fasting program, it may take some time to get into the swing of things. Don't get discouraged! If you slip up, just get back into your intermittent fasting pattern when you can. Avoid beating yourself up, or feeling guilty. Negative self-talk will only prolong you getting back to your pattern. Making a lifestyle change takes a conscious effort, and no one expects you to do it perfectly right away. If you are not used to going long periods without eating, intermittent fasting will take some getting used to. As long as you choose the right method for you, stay focused and remain positive, you will get the hang of it in no time.

Unlike some of the other diet plans that you may go on, the intermittent fast is one that will work. It uses your body and how it works to its advantage to help you to really lose weight. It is easy to get a bit scared when you hear about fasting. You may assume that you need to spend days and weeks without eating (and who really has the willpower to give up their food for that long even when they do want to lose weight) and that it will be too hard for you.

Intermittent fasting is a bit different than you may imagine. Not only is it really hard to go on a fast for weeks at a time, but it is also not good for the body. Your body will often go into starvation mode if you end up being on the fast for too long. It assumes that you are in a time without much food and so the body will work on saving the calories and helping you to hold on to the fat and calories for as long as possible. This means that not only are you hungry, but you are also missing out on losing weight.

You don't have to get too worried about how this intermittent fast will work in the starvation mode. The intermittent fast is effective because you are not going to fast for so long that the body goes into this starvation mode and stops losing weight. Instead, it will make the fast last just long enough that you will be able to speed up the metabolism.

With the intermittent fast, you will find that when you go for a few hours without eating (usually no more than 24ish hours), the body is not going to go right into starvation mode. Rather, it is going to consume the calories that are available. If you ate the right number of calories for the day, the body is going to revert to eating up the stored reserves of fat and use it as fuel. As such, when following an intermittent fasting plan, you force your body to burn more fat without putting in any extra work.

Scientific research on intermittent fasting

You've learned a lot about Intermittent Fasting so far, but you still likely don't understand **why** it all works so well for dieting and health. This chapter is the antidote to that confusion! You will learn how Intermittent Fasting affect the body, how it interacts with diabetes, heart health, aging, and finally, the female body. By the end of this chapter, you should feel both highly informed about IF and aware of a few potential complications.

How IF Affects the Body

When you're feeling hungry, your body is under the sway of two very important hormones: leptin and ghrelin, and Intermittent Fasting affects both of those hormones substantially. In a typical situation, leptin decreases sensations of being hungry, and ghrelin makes you feel hungry instead. While leptin is secreted from fat cells throughout the body, ghrelin is only secreted from the stomach's lining. Together, leptin and ghrelin communicate with the brain's hypothalamus, telling the body when to stop or start eating. During IF, these hormones are released less often, causing the body to have a whole different experience of hunger and fullness.

Another important hormone in the context of eating and hunger suppression is insulin itself. The pancreas produces insulin, and it regulates how much glucose exists in our blood. Ultimately, high or low amounts of insulin affect the individual's weight greatly. Too little insulin and one can't keep weight on. Too much insulin and one can't lose weight whatsoever. While it seems that lower insulin is desired, there has to be a healthy balance, for **too low** insulin is actually disastrous for the body since glucose (or blood sugar) is a large part of how the body gets energy.

One final influencer of the body's hunger and weight loss situation is the individual's thyroid. If the thyroid is overactive, metabolism will work quickly, and energy, health, and weight will be affected. Conversely, an underactive thyroid will slow metabolism, energy, and health, and it will contribute to increased weight.

In the end, Intermittent Fasting affects the individual's weight by varying the production of these three important hormones and by working with the thyroid's natural potential. Essentially, those practicing IF will trigger these hormones to be released less often (or more consistently if the person is obese or diabetic to start with) due to the less-frequent eating schedule.

Eventually, even the thyroid's effects should become balanced out through this altered eating schedule.

IF and Diabetes

For people with diabetes, Intermittent Fasting poses certain risks as well as incredible benefits. People with diabetes have altered insulin levels compared to the non-diabetic person, due to insulin resistance in their bodies. People with Type 1 diabetes cannot make insulin. They need to take insulin daily to have the energy and vigor to live. People with Type 2 diabetes have bodies that don't produce much insulin or don't use that insulin well at all.

With these altered productions of insulin, the blood sugar levels of the body have no way to be regulated, meaning that there's more standing glucose in the blood at all times with no way for it to get into the cells to be used for natural and physical energy. This higher blood sugar level can cause additional problems for the individual over time, but there is no legitimate cure other than taking insulin daily.

Intermittent Fasting, however, can provide a temporary cure when applied correctly in the lives of diabetic individuals (whose diabetic conditions are not severe). When IF is done on a daily basis with just a few fasting hours a day, people with diabetes show improved weight, blood sugar levels, and standing glucose levels. These individuals are not recommended to skip entire meals or fast for days at a time. Also, is not recommended for these people to strictly diet while they're applying IF. Instead, it works better to make food portions smaller and to eat fewer snacks in between.

IF and Heart Health

Heart health is a complicated issue in today's world. We all want to be healthy and thrive, but the foods we eat and the activities we engage in often don't align with those goals, and those more immediate actions win out. In effect, many of our hearts aren't as healthy as they could be. Heart disease is still the biggest killer in the world to this day. However, the introduction of Intermittent Fasting into someone's lifestyle can greatly alter this potential, for it can reduce many risks associated with heart disease.

For example, recent studies done on animals have proved that the practice of Intermittent Fasting improves numerous risk factors for heart disease. Some of these improvements include lowered cholesterol, reduced inflammation in the body, balanced blood sugar levels, and lower blood pressure. Essentially, IF won't cure heart disease, but it will reduce several risk factors that may exist in one's body (with or without him or her knowing).

When it comes down to it, as long as one's Intermittent Fasting experience involves the reintroduction of electrolytes into the body, there's no potential harm posed to the heart whatsoever. There's only potential for growth, bolstering, and strengthening. However, without the right reintroduction of electrolytes, there **is** still the possibility of heart palpitations in individuals attempting IF. The heart needs electrolytes for its stability and efficacy, so as long as you drink a bit of salt with your water, your heart will only thank you!

IF and Aging

People love to talk about how Intermittent Fasting can reverse the effects of aging, and they're not wrong! The tricky part is elucidating the science behind the process they're referencing. The anti-aging potential tied up with Intermittent Fasting applies mostly to two things: 1) your brain and 2) your whole body, through what's called "autophagy."

Overall, Intermittent Fasting heals the body through its ability to rejuvenate the cells. With this restricted caloric intake due to eating schedule or timing, the body's cells can function with less limitation and confusion while producing more energy for the body to use. In effect, the cells function more efficiently while the body can burn more fat and take in more oxygen for the organs and blood, encouraging the individual to live longer with increased sensations of "youth."

About those two original examples, Intermittent Fasting has been proven 1) to keep the brain fit and agile. It improves overall cognitive function and memory capacity as well as cleverness, wit, and quick, clear thinking in the moment. Furthermore, Intermittent Fasting 2) keeps the cells fit and agile through autophagy (which is kick started by IF), where the cells are encouraged to clean themselves up and get rid of any "trash" that might be clogging up the works. By just restricting your eating schedule a little bit each day (or each week), you can find your brain power boosted and your body ready for anything.

IF and the Female Body

Intermittent Fasting requires a different technique than most diets do, which is why it's more often referred to as a lifestyle. Additionally, this variance means that the effects of IF on the female body are a little different than the effects of the standard diet. For instance, dieting will easily cause weight loss in most people, but IF is a little trickier and much less consistent for women especially.

The female body, being created with birthing potential, has specific needs that are altered through an Intermittent Fasting eating schedule. With less hormones being released (which tell women when they are hungry and full), there is less fat being stored in their bodies and less fertility when it comes to their later aims of reproducing. In combination with a strict diet that counts calories or restricts fats, Intermittent Fasting can be dangerous for women of all ages.

For women who still want to work with Intermittent Fasting, there's a lot of hope left for you! Just make sure to follow these four steps to ensure that you're doing it in the most healthy way for your body and your future children. First, make sure you're very connected to your body. You'll want to be very aware if something on the inside seems "off" or "wrong" (bodily, emotionally, and mentally), especially considering all that's at stake, hormonally and reproductively.

 Second, make serious effort to be aware of your body's cycles and note when things go askew. Without the right awareness of your menstruation, you risk going a long time with an altered cycle. This alteration might not sound like a lot, but it can affect many different aspects of your body and your childrearing potential.

Third, please don't try to combine strict dieting and Intermittent Fasting. I know you want to be fit and strong and slim, but you still want to make sure you're getting enough fat and calories, considering what your body is able to do with these right amounts of fat and calories.

Fourth and finally, make sure you're also not exercising too ferociously while you first transition to Intermittent Fasting. If you've been trying IF as a lifestyle for a while, you're welcome to add fitness and exercise back into the mix, but it is really dangerous for the female body to combine two intense practices at once. I understand the urge to lose weight and be healthy, but you'll need to make sure you're not eliminating **too much** from your body at any given time.

Facts About Intermittent Fasting

Although intermittent fasting provides many benefits, it does face some criticism. For example, some people believe that fasting is unsafe because it deprives you of calories, makes you too hungry, or makes it harder to lose weight because your body goes into starvation mode. However, these are all myths as people have been fasting for centuries all over the world to stay healthy. As with any diet, you should consult with your doctor about your dieting plans to ensure that it's appropriate for you.

It Does NOT Include Binge Eating

Many critics claim that dieters will indulge in overeating to try to regain "lost" calories after a fast. This, however, is not true for most people. The goal of fasting is to learn how to control your eating habits so that you consume fewer calories and lose weight. While you may binge eat when hungry on other diets, with intermittent fasting, the goal is to fast and use self-control to remain disciplined. Remember that you can adjust the way you fast to cater to your needs, so if you worry that you might struggle with this, fast for less time at the beginning and gradually increase it, as you get more comfortable.

Starvation

The point of this diet is to train your brain to learn what your body actually needs. When fasting, you're not starving yourself – you are teaching your body that you can go without food for periods of time. Additionally, by gaining control over your eating habits, you can prevent stress-eating, a common coping mechanism. When you have practiced intermittent fasting for a while, you will have a healthier approach to food and will be more likely to eat to nourish your body rather than as a way to deal with your emotions.

Hard to Follow

Some critics worry that this diet will be hard to follow. While this can be true during the first couple of days, keep in mind that this is because you are working on changing the way that your body thinks about food. During these, days, your body will tell you to go get something sweet or to eat more to satisfy your cravings. However, once you become accustomed to the diet, it will become easier because you will have control over your eating habits.

Example with tables and graphs

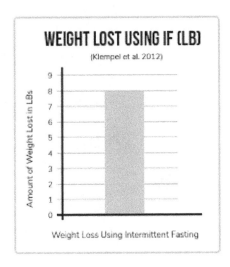

WEIGHT LOST USING IF (LB)

(Klempel et al. 2012)

Amount of Weight Lost in LBs

Weight Loss Using Intermittent Fasting

CHAPTER 5: HOW INTERMITTENT FASTING CAN IMPROVE YOUR LIFE

Benefits of Intermittent Fasting

A number of studies, like those mentioned above, have been done on both humans and animals. These studies evaluated the many benefits of intermittent fasting for controlling weight and other bodily functions. The results have been phenomenal.

Some of the popular health benefits of the IF regimen are:

•   Weight loss: This is the most common health benefit that you can achieve through the intermittent fasting method. You can reduce your belly fat and weight without compromising the calorie intake.

•   Insulin resistance: IF is also capable of decreasing insulin resistance in the body. A follower of this fasting technique will witness a decrease in the levels of insulin by an impressive 20 to 31%. Furthermore, IF reduces the blood sugar levels up to 6%. These figures are enough to protect a person from type 2 diabetes.

•   Inflammation: Much research has revealed a decrease in inflammation markers, which have been noted to be significant catalysts for several chronic diseases.

• Cardiovascular health: IF is known to decrease bad cholesterol levels (LDL) and promote HDL or good cholesterol. In addition, it may decrease the presence of blood triglycerides, which is one of the causes of cardiovascular diseases.

• Cancer: Animals on the IF diet have shown results that display cancer prevention abilities.

• Brain function: IF improves brain function by promoting the growth of nerve cells. Thus, it can help protect against neural disorders, such as Alzheimer's disease.

• Anti-aging properties: IF has been noted to promote longevity in rats, which were part of a fasting experiment. It was found that rats following this diet lived up to 83% longer than rats that weren't on the diet.

Note that while IF may have health benefits, the experiments are still at an initial stage. Several of these studies were conducted for a short duration upon various animals. Therefore, there are still many unanswered questions.

Impact of Intermittent Fasting on Lifestyle

While eating healthy is a simple process, it is not as easy as it seems. One of its primary hurdles is the work needed to cook healthy recipes. However, it does save time by reducing the workload required to prepare several meals a day, thus letting you spend your time doing other things. This makes IF a popular choice among people who prefer life hacks to make their lives easier and healthier. In this way, IF has a significant impact on the lifestyle of an individual.

Intermittent Fasting: Mental Advantages

In addition to physical benefits, IF has mental benefits. This diet plan offers significant benefits related to:

- Boosting memory

- Shielding the mind from neurological disorders such as epilepsy and Alzheimer's disease

- Improving mental focus and clarity

Intermittent Fasting: Enhancing Cognitive Function and Reducing Stress

Intermittent fasting has also shown significant effects with respect to the brain and memory. People who have practiced this diet plan were better able to retain their ability to learn, decreased their oxidative stress, and enhanced their memory.

Many researchers say that this activity takes place because this fasting program manipulates the brain cells to perform more efficiently. During fasting, the cells undergo low/moderate stress, which is why the most efficient cells among them start improvising and adapting to the new condition. This way, the weak cells die, but the stronger ones survive and improve the abilities of the brain.

You can compare it to a high-intensity workout routine at the gym. Exercising is also a type of physical stress that forces your body to endure uncomfortable conditions. As you progress with the regimen, your body starts to adapt to the new conditions, building your muscles, stamina, etc. However, you must rest between your workouts to keep your body ready for the next session.

A similar approach exists when you are practicing IF. Here, your resting intervals will comprise healthy and regular eating sessions, balanced with fasting sessions. That way, you can benefit both your mind and your body.

Thus, you can see that intermittent fasting is capable of improving your cognitive operations due to moderate stress at a cellular level to support and sculpt you.

Additional Benefits of Intermittent Fasting

If you are planning to try intermittent fasting, you will experience the following benefits. Remember that these results will come about only when you are following a strict fasting and eating regimen. IF will help your body achieve the following benefits:

Improves fat loss

If you follow the 16/8 method in which you eat within an eight-hour period and fast for the remaining 16 hours, you can lose a significant amount of weight without having to worry about calories. No doubt, this method will cause the body to lose weight, but those who follow a healthy diet will be able to achieve two times the weight loss than those who prefer junk food will achieve. Thus, through intermittent fasting, you have a way to accomplish your goals, but only when you follow it healthily.

Increases muscle mass

Many people believe that their muscles will fade away while fasting. However, as per research, a 24-hour fast elevated the growth hormone in humans (HGH) up to 1300% for women and 2000% for men. HGH is known for its significance in building muscle cells. With such high numbers, there is a huge effect on the physique of an individual following IF. Increased HGH levels offer enhanced bone mass, increased body mass, and reduced body fat.

Faster recovery

Increased HGH also helps synthesize protein that causes the body to repair and heal faster after an injury or workout session.

Adds suppleness to the skin

With an increase in age, HGH levels decrease. However, during a study, participants who were provided with HGH supplements were found to build muscle and lose fat at a much higher rate. In addition, their skin improved in strength, making it more resistant to wrinkles and sagging.

Reduces the rate of aging

With fasting, your body starts producing stem cells at a much faster rate. These stem cells can be manipulated to become any cell in the body. Therefore, they can replace damaged and old cells, keeping your body younger at the cellular level. These stem cells can help with chronic pain, old injuries, joints, skin, etc. Therefore, instead of going for stem cell therapy, which can be costly, your other option is to focus on intermittent fasting.

Enhances brain functions

Through fasting, you can improve your brain. When you fast, your brain starts generating a protein known as BNF, which is a very crucial building block. This protein helps improve memory and learning power.

In addition, it helps develop complex and robust neural networks to keep the brain functioning smoothly and speedily. This is necessary to keep the brain functions active as you get older.

Triggers autophagy

This process may sound cruel for the cells in your body, but it is of crucial importance. New and strong cells eat away damaged and old cells to make space for fresh and strong ones. This is like a tune-up operation for your body; it will keep the body running smoothly and promote longevity. Through intermittent fasting, the process of autophagy can be triggered.

Reduces inflammation

IF reduces inflammation markers and oxidative stress. Inflammation is responsible for diseases, aging, and poor performance of the body, which is why it must be reduced or eliminated. Preventing inflammation will help the body function more efficiently with increased longevity. IF offers you an upgrade that helps your body adapt to new and tougher conditions, ultimately enhancing your resistance and endurance for your eating habits. The result is a stronger, more efficient body that works on less energy.

Improve immune system

Aside from what it is capable of doing to your overall level of hunger, the ketogenic state is known to dramatically reduce the likelihood of numerous major health issues, starting with all of the types of cancer that are known to feed on glucose directly. While healthy cells can easily switch to burning ketones for energy, cancer cells are not that lucky which means they grow significantly more slowly than they otherwise would when deprived of their primary food source.

Switching to the keto diet is also ideal when it comes to promoting brain health for several reasons. The most important of these is the fact that following the keto diet is closer to the way early humans likely ate which means it is more in line with the type of fuel that the brain is naturally used to consuming. This, in turn, makes it possible for the brain to continue working at maximum capacity for longer than would otherwise be the case.

While it's true that the brain requires glucose to work properly, this is definitely the case of potentially having too much of a good thing. In this instance, if the brain receives too much glucose on a regular basis, then over time it will develop a higher tolerance which means that it will need to work harder in order to generate the same results. If left untreated this can lead to a state of glucose deprivation, which can eventually lead to dementia. Utilizing glycerol as a replacement for glucose can then make it easier for the brain to function in the long-term without having to worry about these types of adverse effects; meaning that it is far more likely that degradation will occur.

Reduces inflammation

Inflammation, which is a fundamental cause of many common diseases, can be reduced by intermittent fasting.

Inflammation is likely the biggest negative influence on all poor health conditions, whether physical or mental. Acute inflammation is a positive thing, as it essentially tells the body there is an issue that requires immediate attention. This triggers cells to jump into action, rebuild, and repair. Think of it like going out for a run—the exercise makes your muscles sore, but because of that exercise, your cells rebuild and come back stronger. Without that activity and soreness, there is no opportunity to become stronger. The problem comes when that inflammation does not dissipate due to constant exposure to physical and mental stressors such as money, drama, kids, work deadlines, pollution, chemicals, and over-processed foods. While we cannot rid our lives of stress, we can help the body react more positively to that stress. Intermittent fasting has been shown to reduce C-reactive protein and cytokines, internal markers of stress. Giving your body a break from constantly consuming food allows it to target and care for areas outside the digestive system.

CHAPTER 6: POTENTIAL SIDE EFFECTS

Feeling hungry

You Will Always be Hungry

There will be times when you will feel hungry when you first get started. Just stick with it for a couple of weeks, and once that first week is done, it will be much easier. Eventually, you will have trained yourself to respond to hunger when it's time to eat, instead of as a reaction to cravings and hunger pains.

Intermittent fasting is not something that is impossible to follow and there are some basic principles to help guide you. For example, instead of trying to change everything about your diet from quantity to food selection, this diet instead focuses on changing *when* you eat while controlling your total calories.

Hormonal imbalance

When you do not eat for some time, several things happen to your body. For example, your body will start initiating processes for cell repair and change some of your hormone levels, which makes stored body fat easier to access.

Constipation

Constipation is related to Bloating, and it's just one of those things that might happen in your body as you get used to eating less or at incredibly different times than normal. Remember to drink a lot of water so whatever **is** in your system has enough hydration to come out without stress. Within a few weeks, the water cure (drink A LOT!!!) should help flush out the issue.

Irritability

This is one of the most commonly unexpected side-effects from Intermittent Fasting, but it is very prevalent, especially for people just beginning to transition into the lifestyle. People get angry! It's a thing. People get snippy and sassy when they're waiting for food. Unfortunately, this will be you, but you're definitely going to learn a lot about yourself during this period, and you'll eventually grow **through** these irritable feelings. Be patient with yourself (and especially patient with others). The irritability will fade, I promise.

Feeling cold

Is another of those things none of us would likely expect from practicing Intermittent Fasting. You will probably feel extra sensitive to the cold through your fingers and toes while you're fasting, but this side-effect is totally normal! Don't be alarmed when you feel it. Instead, just know that it means your body is burning fat and your blood sugar is decreasing, and these effects are standard and healthy to experience. Drink a little extra hot tea or wear a few extra layers to help keep warm.

Heartburn

Is a more uncommon side-effect of Intermittent Fasting, but it's another thing that's totally natural. Your stomach is used to producing acids to digest the foods you're consuming, and when you start adjusting to IF, these acids are being produced at times when you're potentially fasting, causing heartburn or reflux issues. With time, this side-effect should be mitigated if not totally alleviated. Keep drinking water and try not to eat foods that are super greasy or spicy when you do breakfast. If things don't get better, consider speaking with your doctor or nutritionist.

Bloating

Is a side-effect related to #5 above, Constipation. When you transition into Intermittent Fasting, your stomach is going to be processing things in a way that it hasn't in a long, long time— possibly ever. There will be weird side-effects like this for some, but it's all part of that adjustment period, and these issues should resolve themselves in a week or so. Drink a lot of water to aid the situation!

More frequent urination

Is common as well, and this situation most often arises due to the displacement of eating for the sake of the fast. During these fast periods, individuals are invited to drink anything (that doesn't have too many calories), and this often translates to a full bladder almost constantly—at least in the beginning! When things get tough, you'll want to drink more water. If things get gurgle-y or constipated on the inside, you'll want to drink more water. If you have headaches or get lightheaded, you'll want some water with a pinch of salt. If you need energy, you'll grab the coffee. You get the picture. Expect frequent bathroom runs.

CHAPTER 7: TYPES OF INTERMITTENT FASTING DIET

Different Types of Intermittent Fasting

12-hour fast

For women unsure of where to begin, the Crescendo method, or 12/12 plan, is a great place to start and is best for those who need a lot of flexibility, because you can eat from 7 a.m. to 7 p.m. one day and 10 a.m. to 10 p.m. the next. As long as the periods between eating last at least 12 hours, you are doing it right. Freelancers, women with young children, and athletes might be more compatible with this fasting approach. Women who are currently feeling burned out or run down, or dealing with hormonal imbalances are advised to slowly work their way into the full 12 hours. Instead of going all-in tomorrow, take a few weeks to ease into it. For example, this week, simply track when you naturally stop eating (snacks, alcohol, etc.) and when you reach for your first bite in the morning. The next week, commit to fasting for eight hours every day of the week. This should be simple because you will mostly be sleeping during the fast. For the third week, extend your fast to 10 hours, and finally get to 12 hours after a month of easing into the process. Letting your body slowly adjust to fasting will help you understand which time schedule works best for you, keep you from feeling overwhelmed, and will allow your body's hormones and metabolic processes to adapt.

On this plan, it is important to define your fasting windows in order to be accountable and committed. As I mentioned earlier, they come with a lot of flexibility, but you still have to define them. Think about your daily work schedule and exercise times and how they will be impacted by your choice. Most women will find success consuming calories earlier in the day, as their bodies burn fat slowly and tend to have finicky digestive systems compared to males. Women also tend to crave more sweets, which leads to overeating in the evening. Ending the eating window several hours before going to bed will help improve digestion, promote an efficient metabolism, and prevent snacking on unneeded sweets at a time they're more likely to be stored as fat. This plan should help you tune in to your hunger levels, circadian rhythm, and work to naturally reset and refine habits.

16/8

This is the second most adopted method of IF by women. The 16/8 intermittent fasting method is a time-restricted way of promoting weight loss. You eat in an 8-hour window in a day and fast for the remaining 16 hours. Let us be clearer about what this window can be, and how you fast for those long 16 hours.

You can stop eating at 7 p.m., skip the morning breakfast and start again by 11 a.m. The 11-7 window is your time to eat.

Or, you can have breakfast and lunch and skip dinner.

Your meals should focus on high nutritional value. If you think you can eat burgers and pizzas during your eight-hour window, you would not achieve much from this diet. You can take unsweetened drinks like water, black coffee and tea during the fasting period.

Please remember that your body will need some time to adjust to the new routine. You are likely to feel dizzy and nauseated in the beginning for at least a week. You might experience binge-eating tendencies to give up and start eating. But, once your body accepts your eating pattern, this fasting method can work beautifully for you.

5/2

The 5:2 method is about what and when you eat. This method means that you'll eat regularly for five days a week, but then have two days where you eat a drastically reduced calorie diet.

While most people eat roughly 2,200 calories in a day, while you're on the 5:2 fast, you'll eat your 2,200 calories for five days, but then eat only 500-600 calories on the two fasting days.

The benefits of having the calorie restriction twice per week means that you are more likely to lose weight, even if you overeat slightly on the days when you follow your normal diet. The 5:2 diet hasn't been more heavily researched than many other kinds of intermittent fasting, but what has been researched shows some promising studies about it. While many studies are with animals as subjects, there are a few with human participants too.

In some of the studies, it is believed that the 5:2 method can reduce tumors in breast cancer and help with other physiological issues in the body. It can help improve insulin resistance and prevent cardiovascular disease. While these studies are promising, just keep in mind that many of them revolved around animals. You can find the studies in the reference page at the end of this book, if you would like to do further research.

In general, the 5:2 method can provide you with weight loss that is on par with people who reduce calories every day. However, some people find reducing calories everyday to be very restrictive. After all, there's only so much you can eat on a calorie restrictive diet. However, with the 5:2 method, you can eat whatever you want for your eating days, and only reduce your calories on your fasting day. While you can eat whatever you want, you should still maintain a well-balanced diet. Eating only junk food won't help with your weight loss goals, if that is the reason you're choosing to fast.

While the 5:2 method can be very beneficial, some people struggle with their first few fast days. After eating 2,000 calories on day one, followed by 500 calories on day two, you can feel almost uncontrollably hungry. However, many people say (anecdotally) that the hunger fades if you keep yourself distracted. Furthermore, so long as you follow the fast for a while, you'll soon no longer feel hungry during your fast days. All of this is anecdotal of course, but it is something to consider when choosing to fast with the 5:2 method.

Alternative days

Alternative Day fasting is like an extended version of the 5:2 method. There's actually a lot of research that supports alternate day fasting, and it's considered to be really good for reducing belly fat in people who are very obese. Even if weight is maintained, there's a good chance that alternate day fasting can lead to better health overall. It can reduce insulin levels and insulin resistance and can help the brain handle cell stress (Anson et al., 2003). There are a lot of studies about it, but as mentioned before, some of these studies are animal studies. However, they provide some promising implications for how alternate day fasting can help humans.

In this fast, you are fasting every other day, and eating your regular portions on your off days. This means that you have an overall reduced calorie load during the week. This is similar to a regular calorie reduction diet, where calories are reduced everyday. So, the weekly calorie restriction can be the same in both the fast and the diet. However, people generally find alternate day fasting easier to follow than calorie restricted diets. There are some people who dislike the alternate day fast because it can be very difficult to go hungry during the fasting days. This hunger doesn't always get easier as the weeks go on. This can strain people's motivation to continue the fast. Some people combat this by eating a reduced calorie meal on fasting days. In this case, this adaptation makes the alternate day fast like the 5:2 fast, with just extra days of fasting.

Because there is a significant calorie reduction, it's important that the meals you eat are nutritious. You don't want to be undernourished while following this fast. Additionally, if you're already at a healthy weight, this fast may make you lose weight that you can't afford to lose. So be careful when approaching this fast. However, if you are very overweight, then this fast can help you. Just work with your doctor to figure out if this fast will be of benefit to you. As mentioned earlier, there is significant research associated with alternate day fasting, and a lot of it is positive. So, this style of fasting can bring you significant benefits.

To conclude this chapter, there are several different options for following an intermittent fast. You should choose the fasting method that works for you and your lifestyle. If you're a very social eater, then choose a fast like the 14:10 fast or perhaps the 5:2 fast. If you're very determined, have great discipline, and can maintain motivation, then choose a fast like the 24-hour, alternate day, or the Warrior Diet. Either way, you'll likely get some benefits from these fast choices. However, with benefits, always come risks. These fasts all have some risks associated, and it's important to know them before choosing to follow intermittent fasting. In the next chapter, we'll be discussing the benefits of fasting in general, and explore the risks associated with fasting.

CHAPTER 8: PRACTICAL GUIDE TO INTERMITTENT FASTING: FROM BEGINNER TO EXPERT

Guide to start intermittent fasting and to become an expert

Get tuned in, to your body

This is key. No one knows your own body but yourself. Be alert for signs of threats to your health. If blood glucose regulation (i.e., diabetes) is a problem, consult a doctor first before considering intermittent fasting.

Fasting should not be done in such extremes as totally starving the body. This could lead to more serious problems in the long run. If there is a craving or intense need to feed during a fasting period, eat. This is not a rigid dieting program. One can always adjust the fast/feed schedule.

Track your progress

Nothing is more encouraging than seeing your body get in better shape and see the fruits of your efforts. Regularly evaluate the body's response to this program. It helps with encouraging one to go on, or to assess if the program works or if it is already harmful.

Discipline yourself

While this is not a strict weight loss program, keep the amount of food you eat in check. Avoid overcompensating food intake during normal days. It is OK to eat a little during fast periods, but remember to adjust on succeeding meals.

Make healthy food choices

Normal days do not mean an eat-all-you-can binge session. Consume only within the required daily calorie needs. Choose foods that have an overall healthy benefit. Occasional indulgences on sweet and calorie-rich foods are acceptable. Remember not to overindulge.

Relax and enjoy the process

This is most probably the most enjoyable, and easiest to adhere to, among the weight loss programs. No special diets, no particular food restrictions, and no rigid eating schedule. No need to freak out if the daily fast period is less than 16 hours. Beverages need not be restricted to no-calorie ones. Practitioners of intermittent fasting can choose from a wide array of regular food. Just enjoy eating, in moderation.

Choosing the right plan

There are many methods of intermittent fasting. In the end, the only one you should choose is one that is going to work for you. Perhaps the hardest part about reaping the benefits of IF is that you are going to be hungrier than usual at the start. Stick with it! Sticking with IF may mean trying many different IF methods until you find one that you like. This doesn't mean finding an IF method that isn't any struggle at all, but rather finding an IF method that you know you can keep up with for whatever amount of time you've set as your goal. If your goal is to use IF to lose fat in 90 days, choose a plan that *you can stick with for 90 days*.

108

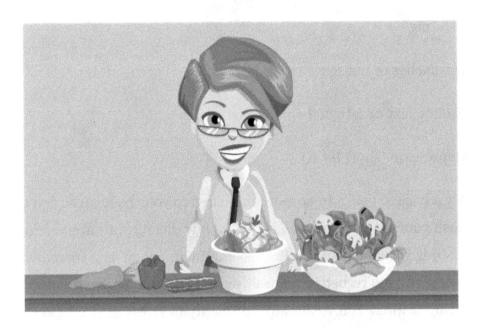

Women's bodies have built-in mechanisms that prevent losing fat. Evolutionarily speaking, it would protect your reproductive abilities, which is dependent on keeping those precious fat stores. It's just something you'll have to deal with. It's certainly not impossible to do though.

For women, fasting is a slightly different animal all together because women have more sensitivity to hunger hormones and they need to deal with more complicated reproductive processes. These may cause troubles that will affect your ability to fast. Some signs you're experiencing hormonal imbalance during fasting:

Irregular periods

Bloating

Headaches or nausea

Feeling lazy or fatigued

Depression (short term)

My advice to you is to go slow and listen to your body. Just don't push yourself too hard and let your body dictate your approach. Also, if you are planning to become pregnant or are currently pregnant, you're better off waiting until well after birth before trying fasting. You've already got plenty of stress as it is! Don't add to it with attempting to fast. Besides, IF can mess with cycles and fertility, so learn your body's tolerance to fasting first. I've read that it shouldn't affect the child if you're already fully fat adapted, but listen to your body and your doctor. Ultimately, IF should be improving your life, not making it worse. If it just doesn't work for you, then listen to your body and slowly make small changes.

Fasting is NOT anorexia.

One major piece of advice for women especially: Don't let fasting turn into anorexia. Fasting is not about starving yourself; it's about eating naturally and optimizing your health. If you're barely eating ~1000 calories a day for long term, your body will begin to waste away and it will cause damage over time. You need to see food as something to keep your body going strong and healthy, not something to be completely avoided or mindlessly indulged. Alternate day fasts or multi-day fasts can be beneficial, but there comes a point where the benefits taper off and you're just hurting yourself. Anorexia is a slippery slope; don't let it happen to you.

Besides, *barely eating anything is the worst possible way to lose weight and look good.* Anorexia would only end up with muscle wasting and hampered fat burning, as well as psychological damage. This is seen in the results of the "**Minnesota starvation experiment.**" If you truly want to lose *only fat*, keto can help to burn the fat and IF can help to keep it off. From there, it's all about finding your ideal weight and maintaining it with good food and exercise. If you starve yourself, you'll look and feel miserable, plus you won't have any energy. It's all about the protein, just keep it high enough to keep your muscles and only fat will be burned. Roughly .4-.6 grams of protein per kg will be fine for non-weightlifters, and at least 1-2 grams per kg for weight lifting. Just check the nutritional facts and do the math. (Moreover, no; meat won't kill **you** like the media claims.)

They're called "essential amino acids" for a reason!

This is why I don't recommend a vegan/vegetarian diet as well; there's just not enough protein and many people waste away on those diets. Animal fats and proteins are far better for our bodies than plant based versions, thanks to the bioavailability/absorption of those macronutrients. We just can't utilize the broken down parts of a plant as well as an animal.

I have met numerous people who are ex-vegetarians that gave up the diet because it decimated their minds and bodies, while switching to a paleo-based diet was able to keep the weight off and allow the body to function properly. *We're animals, we need other animals to survive and thrive.* If you still have any ethical concerns, my suggestion is to reduce your store-bought meats and support your local farms. Pasture raised chickens and 100% grass fed cows are far happier and healthier than the mass-produced meats from the mega-grocery stores.

The Health Benefits Of Intermittent Fasting For Women

Intermittent fasting not only benefits your waist, but can also reduce the risk of developing several chronic diseases.

Heart health

Heart disease is the leading cause of death worldwide

High blood pressure, high LDL cholesterol, and high triglyceride concentrations are among the leading risk factors for cardiovascular disease.

One study involving 16 men and women with obesity showed that intermittent fasting reduced blood pressure by 6% in just eight weeks.

In the same study, it was also found that intermittent fasting lowers LDL cholesterol by 25% and triglycerides by 32%.

However, data on the relationship between intermittent fasting and increased levels of LDL cholesterol and triglycerides do not agree.

A study with 40 people with normal weight showed that four weeks of intermittent fasting during the Islamic holiday of Ramadan does not lead to a decrease in LDL cholesterol or triglycerides.

Better studies with more reliable methods are needed before researchers can fully understand the effect of intermittent fasting on heart health.

Diabetes

Intermittent fasting can also effectively help manage and reduce the risk of developing diabetes.

Like constant calorie restriction, intermittent fasting seems to reduce certain risk factors for diabetes.

This is mainly due to a decrease in insulin levels and a decrease in insulin resistance.

However, intermittent fasting may not be as beneficial for women as it is for men in terms of blood sugar levels.

A small study showed that blood sugar control worsened in women after a 22-day fast, while in men, the fast did not hurt blood sugar levels.

Despite this side effect, a decrease in insulin resistance is likely to reduce the risk of developing diabetes, especially for people with pre-diabetes.

Weight loss

Intermittent fasting can be a simple and effective way to lose weight if done correctly, as regular short-term posts can help you consume fewer calories and lose pounds.

Several studies show that intermittent fasting is just as effective as traditional calorie-restricted diets for short-term weight loss.

A review of studies conducted in 2018 for overweight adults showed that intermittent fasting resulted in an average weight loss of 15 pounds (6.8 kg) for 3–12 months.

Another review showed that intermittent fasting reduced body weight by 3–8% in adults with overweight or obesity for 3–24 weeks. The survey also showed that participants reduced waist size by 3–7% over the same period.

It should be noted that the long-term effect of intermittent fasting on weight loss in women remains to be seen.

In the short term, intermittent hunger seems to help in weight loss. However, the amount you lose is likely to depend on the number of calories you consume during periods without fasting, and how long you keep your lifestyle.

It can help you eat less

Going on intermittent fasting can, of course, helps you eat less.

One study found that young people ate 650 calories less per day when their food intake was limited to a four-hour interval.

Another study conducted on 24 healthy men and women was devoted to studying the effect of a long 36-hour fast on eating habits. Despite the consumption of extra calories in post-post day, participants reduced the total calorie balance by 1,900 calories, which is a significant reduction.

The Nutritional Needs of Women

There are many ways fasting and weight-loss recommendations apply to both men and women; however, women have some unique needs, meaning that a few female-specific modifications should be made. Understanding your physiology will help you target your needs and obtain your goals faster. Let's explore several important nutritional needs in more detail so you can feel confident in your approach to better your health throughout this process.

Calcium: While many bodily functions involve this mineral, including heart and nerve regulation, its bone-strengthening aspect is most relevant to women. As we age, estrogen production declines, and bone loss accelerates, putting women at greater risk of brittle bones and osteoporosis. To promote

116

your health, rely on whole foods like dairy and leafy greens rather than calcium supplements. Consuming enough vitamin D is also needed to properly absorb calcium in foods.

Magnesium: This mighty mineral is involved in over 600 bodily functions, including enhancing energy metabolism and promoting sleep quality, according to one comprehensive study. Additional research says that it also fights inflammation, high insulin levels, and accelerated aging. Magnesium levels tend to fall throughout the menstrual cycle and should be a focus of any woman's healthful diet.

Folate: According to at least one research study, this mineral directly supports a healthy pregnancy because it prevents neural tube defects in developing infants. Additionally, the Centers for Disease Control recommends all prenatal women, regardless of plans for future pregnancy, get enough of this nutrient. Even if you aren't motivated by reproductive reasons, getting enough folate from sources such as greens, citrus, nuts, seeds, or fortified foods can help your body burn carbohydrates.

Iron: Red blood cells need iron to carry oxygen to tissues and muscles throughout the body. When iron stores become low, the body becomes fatigued due to the inability to transport oxygen. Recommendations say women should take 18 grams a day. This is because you lose iron through menstruation. When you're not fasting, you'll want to focus on consuming iron-rich foods. While many foods contain iron, the body has a very hard time absorbing it from food, and for this reason, a supplement might be worthwhile.

Vitamin C: Your body needs this super vitamin to help absorb more of the iron you eat. Your best bet is to eat it at every meal by consuming healthful fruits and vegetables loaded with this nutrient. Vitamin C also helps skin stay radiant and youthful.

B12: This nutrient plays a large role in energizing your body and revving up your metabolism because of its vital function in processing the macronutrients protein and fat, which can affect achieving your body goals. This nutrient is found in animal products, meaning vegetarians or vegans will need a supplement.

Thiamine: Also known as B1, this compound is essential for carbohydrate metabolism. Consuming enough thiamine will help your metabolism stay high and enable your body to process the foods you consume more efficiently. Foods rich in this vitamin include potatoes, kale, eggs, and many fortified grain products.

While every nutrient—macronutrients, phytonutrients, vitamins, and minerals—is vital to health, paying more attention to those listed here can support your health and metabolism while fasting. During non-fasting periods, consume a balanced, nutrient-rich diet to prevent any deficiencies or fatigue.

The Science of the Human Body

Have you ever wondered why it happens to be that you eat more when you're hungry than you're hungry for? Have you ever been curious about why you sometimes can't stop even when you know you're full? As someone coming to IF with goals of weight loss, you likely are very familiar with these frustrating feelings, but if you're coming to IF with goals other than weight loss, you might not be as familiar.

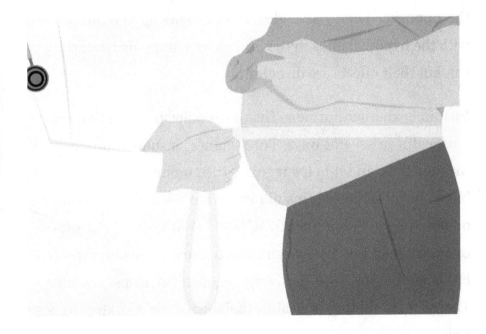

Regardless of your experience with hunger and whether or not you're able to stop eating when you feel you're full, there are scientific reasons why the saying "Your eyes were bigger than your stomach" exists. First on this list of reasons is the existence of hormones leptin and ghrelin. Both leptin and ghrelin seem to have a large effect on regulating appetite, and subsequently controlling fat storage and gain.

While leptin is secreted from fat cells in the stomach, heart, skeletal muscle, and placenta in females, ghrelin is secreted basically only from the lining of the stomach. Despite where the hormones come from, however, they both end up affecting the brain. Leptin decreases feelings of hunger, while ghrelin does the opposite. Leptin and ghrelin both end up communicating with the hypothalamus in the brain about stopping or starting to eat, but their effects are divergent.

Insulin is another hormone that our bodies produce that effects our health in several ways. For instance, insulin is produced in the pancreas, and it helps regulate the amount of glucose in our blood, but if someone's insulin levels are too high or too low, his or her weight is imminently affected. With low insulin levels, one can't help but lose weight, but too low of insulin levels can be dangerous because the body needs sugar to use as energy. The trick is finding a healthy balance while working to lose weight.

If you're overweight or working with IF, your hormones' signals to the brain become affected. If you're obese, for instance, the signals are interrupted and distorted, while for those working with IF, those signals are triggered not to go off as frequently through an altered pattern of eating.

One final element to note in this section would be the thyroid, whose function is essential in determining both health and ability with weight loss. The thyroid regulates hormones that affect the speed of your metabolism, and if your thyroid is over- or under-worked, your health, energy level, and weight will certainly be affected. In order to lose weight, you'll want to speed up your metabolism without hurting or overworking your thyroid, and that can be tricky to work out properly sometimes.

How the Male vs. Female Bodies React to Hunger

When it comes to the science of the human body, everything matters, from the foods we eat to how often we eat, what hormones we allow to produce, which ones we limit, and how well our thyroids are working.

When you're hungry, your body sends signals to the vagus nerve in your brain, and it communicates a lot of details. It reveals how empty (or full) your stomach happens to be, the nutrients that are processed in the intestines, and what deficiencies may be present in the body as a whole. After the stomach sits empty, it starts to grumble (a process called "borborygmus," which pushes any remaining food into the intestines to be digested fully), and then your stomach and intestinal walls begin producing that hormone, ghrelin, that makes you feel hungry.

If you're female and you tell yourself you're not hungry when you get this feeling, your brain often doesn't work in your favor. The hypothalamus and vagus nerve get triggered, making you feel hungry even if you keep telling yourself you can't eat yet or aren't mentally hungry. In the male body, however, the physical hunger sensations and hormone secretions can be limited in effect to the brain through inhibitive thoughts against hunger and eating.

Furthermore, a study on female versus male rats from 2013 revealed that when females (opposed to males) fast for a few days at a time, their abilities to control that hunger response become more fine-tuned than males' do, leading to their ability to lose more weight overall than the male rats could. This study clearly applies to humans' experiences with intermittent fasting as well.

Reasons for Sex Distinction with IF

The primary reason why there is a separation of males and females in the study regarding IF is that the reproductive organs of males and females are different, making their responses to intermittent fasting dissimilar. With different reproductive organs and different reproductive capacities, these two sexes will have different sets of hormones being produced at different times and being sent to very diverse spaces in the body.

Ultimately, it is true that these two sexes will have different responses to fasting, in terms of weight loss potential and reproductive health. As the rat study from 2013 reminds us, females can lose weight faster through IF than males can, but they also have restricted abilities to have children during those times of IF (while males don't), which absolutely reaffirms the importance of sex distinction in studies of (and practice with) intermittent fasting in the human world. Different bodies respond differently to things that jolt the system like IF, and it's truer to say that each person's process with IF will be dissimilar. However, the first step is making distinctions based on sex and hormonal realities so that the individual comes out of the fast as healthy and energetic as possible.

When it comes down to it, noting sex differences, as it pertains to weight loss work with fasting, helps refine the process of IF for the individual. With these differences taken into account and planned for, the results of the fasting lifestyle change are better, meaning more productive, less restricting, and more beneficial for the health of the individual overall.

CHAPTER 11: INTERMITTENT FASTING FOR PEOPLE 50+

There is one thing you need to keep in mind about intermittent fasting when you are over 50: your metabolism. As you age, your metabolism slows down. As a result, you will become slower and your body requires fewer calories to maintain itself. That means you can cut down on calories in greater quantity than you did in your twenties.

If you are just starting out and are wondering whether intermittent is for you, then you could try out fast-mimicking first. Fast mimicking is a modified fasting regimen that allows you to consume a certain amount of calorie while still allowing you to get the benefits of fasting.

This type of fasting generally lasts for about five days and you need to keep your carb, protein, and calorie intake low while keeping your fat intake high. Your calories should be kept at roughly 40% of your ordinary intake. This means you would still be nourished with electrolytes and nutrients.

The best thing about fast mimicking is the fact that it is easier on the body than traditional fasting or intermittent fasting. So, how do you do fast mimicking?

The whole idea behind mimic fasting is to trick your body into thinking that you are fasting. That way, your body responds accordingly, and you can get all of those benefits of fasting while you still continue to nourish your body.

You do not need to do it for long, either. Most of the time, you only need to do it between 3 and 7 days. As always, make sure you consult your doctor first before you commit to this.

To begin, ask yourself whether you are interested in tracking your fasting outcomes. If so, then consider measuring certain biomarkers such as blood glucose, ketones, and weight change on a daily basis, in addition to doing lab tests before and after your fast.

It also helps if you set up an environment conducive for your fasting effort. You can do so by:

- Letting those you plan on seeing while you are fasting know what you are doing and why it is important for you, so you can get emotional support.
- Taking away temptations such as snacks at home and work.
- Sleeping more, because you will be more tired than usual.
- Planning for some exercise each day, but stick to the light, easy exercises.

- Creating a meal plan so you know what you put into your body.

It is recommended to start off your first fasting-mimicking day by eating 50% of your usual daily calorie intake as opposed to the 40% we mentioned earlier. That way, your body can adjust. From the second day to the fifth, you can then gradually work toward the target 35% to 40% of the intake. You should also eat something that your body can digest easily.

While there is a pre-packed fast mimicking diet called ProLon FMD that contains all five days' worth of food for the fast, you do not need to go out of your way to buy it. Just make sure you match the numbers and plan your meals properly. The numbers are:

First day: 34% carbs, 10% protein, and 56% fat.

Remaining days: 47% carbs, 9% protein, and 44% fat.

Note: The percentage represents a portion of the calorie intake. That means 1,000kcal for women and 1,250kcal for men for the first day. For the remaining days, it is 800kcal for women and 1,000kcal for men.

Other than that, if you love coffee or tea, then you can drink either a cup of black coffee or tea per day. If you do, make sure they do not contain any added creams or sugar.

CHAPTER 12: HOW TO COMBINE INTERMITTENT FASTING WITH SPORT & FITNESS

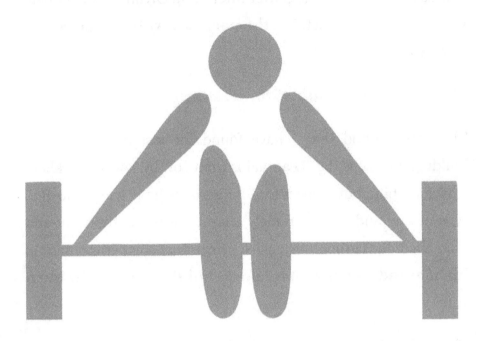

If you are a woman

You might be surprised to learn that exercising while fasting can provide a host of different benefits. In fact, it can actually be more beneficial than eating before exercise! Plus, once a person is used to being fully fasted and fat-adapted, there's actually **very little active energy lost when exercising on an empty stomach**

Fasting makes exercise easier

Unless you're a high-end power lifter or an Olympic level athlete with a very specific diet, **it's the perfect way to supercharge your workouts.**

It's called "Lean-Gains" for a reason!

The best method that I have found for losing weight while building muscle is the "Lean-gains protocol" by Martin Berkhan. I have nothing but respect for him because he is truly a no-B.S. type of guy and he's extremely smart. He walks the walk and talks the talk. Through extensive research and experimentation, **his method can simultaneously build muscle AND burn fat.**

If you glazed over at all when reading about hormones, prepare to be totally confused and put to sleep.

Supercharge your fat loss!

It's certainly not easy but it's worth the effort if you can do it. Even if you can't follow it to a T, it's still a great way to exercise. Here's the cool thing about a fasted workout: *You're combining the enhanced fat burning of fasting along with the exercise releasing additional compounds and hormones that will cause even more fat burning.* Plus, in the case of weight lifting, you're burning calories as you repair your muscles over the course of 2-3 days, **so the fat loss effect is truly "supercharged!"** You can literally burn fat just from sitting around thanks to your muscles being repaired.

For those of you who weight-lift, I would strongly suggest looking into **Branched chain amino acids (BCAA's)**. The science behind them is fairly complicated, but **it's essential for any serious fasting weight lifter**. The major benefit is that it is able to provide the amino acids required for muscle repair, but it also won't kill the fasted state like most other supplements. By maintaining the fasted state along with a strenuous weight-based workout, you can really supercharge your fat burning and simultaneously build muscle better than a normal weight lifter. This is because the strenuous training will increase the fat burning via the adrenaline release, which will trigger fatty acid release from fat stores. You can also use carbs in a way that makes them build more muscle. For almost every other exercise, you're good to go.

For those of you who don't weight lift on a regular basis, you really don't need food before most typical non weight-based workouts.

Exercising while fasted can activate the following benefits:

- Enhanced insulin sensitivity (which will help make fasting easier overall)
- Build muscle quicker and more efficiently
- Improve recovery time (with BCAA supplementation)
- Better lifting via muscle glycogen retention and repletion
- Improved adaption to exercise

No matter what your end goal is, exercise more. If you can, do it on an empty stomach. Period. Just be sure to drink plenty of water!

If you are a man

As you consider getting started with ketogenic diet and intermittent fasting, there are key factors that should be put into consideration. You should ensure that you stay within the macros for keto diet as you also eat enough calories during the eating period. Fasting should be combined with optimal nutrition; sufficient sleep, and work with reduced stress if the desired benefits are to be realized. If you find the two to be challenging, then you can begin with ketogenic diet and get keto adapted before incorporating intermittent fasting.

When you are getting started, it's likely that the body is still dependent on intake of high carbs and utilization of glucose so you are likely to feel hungry much faster which makes it difficult to stick with fasting. Once the body adapts to ketosis where ketones are seen as the source of energy, fasting then feels more natural and manageable. Starting the process gradually helps people to adapt well to the process, unlike jumping into change at once. You can begin the process by cutting on the regular intake of snacks, then gradually move to cutting full meals.

Finding your macros is vital as you get started since you need to decide the number of calories, proteins, carbs, and fats that you should be eating each day. If you goal is to lose weight then defining your macros is a critical step. Once you have set the number of macros, you should then commit to eating the set amount of macronutrients. If your intention is to lose weight, then a lot of emphasis should be given to sticking with the required number of macros.

It's important that you consume all the calories during the eating window as you also follow the approved intake of keto foods to ensure that your body stays on ketosis. There are endless options of healthy and nutritious ketogenic diet foods that you can choose from, but you have to decide to do away with high carbohydrate foods. Before the body adapts to high fat diet, there will instances where you get to experience serious hunger cravings as you engage in intermittent fasting. Just ensure that you avoid any form of binging on carbs so that you don't get thrown out of ketosis.

During the feeding period, the number of meals that one gets to consume doesn't actually matter; all that matters is maintaining the caloric intake which should constitute the macronutrients and the calories that one gets to consume. If you want 1000 calories per day then you should ensure that you consume all the calories during the eating window. As a beginner, you can decide to maintain a wider feeding window like 8 hours within the day but that should reduce as you get acquainted with the fasting process and keto diet.

As the body gets accustomed to fasting and keto diet, you should also be able to make the feeding window shorter for improved benefits. You can opt to skip breakfast then have some good lunch and dinner. Keep testing how short you can make the feeding window to be before your body begins to resist.

Being on ketogenic diet and intermittent fasting puts the body into a prime primal state where one is completely self-sufficient and also capable of producing energy regardless of the time and the number of calories that one gets to consume. It's possible to fail even with the combination if you lack insight on what goes on psychologically and how you can sustain the process. When one is getting started, it's more likely that the body is not on ketosis and that's why it's vital that they take time and go through a period of keto-adaptation.

If you get started when the body is still geared towards burning sugar for fuel then it might take such a longer time before you get into ketosis state and the side effects might be very intense. Fasting on keto should follow several stages for the adaptation to take place.

The Plan to Build the Ultimate Body

The correct training, nutrition and dedication to follow a tough training schedule designed to shock the muscles into growth can yield fantastic results. Now combine that with Intermittent Fasting and you move into a whole new world of gaining muscle and leaning up.

Do you want to move to the next level of physical performance?

1 - Training Frequency

Many people say you can only train a body part once a week. This theory is fast becoming outdated and obsolete. All we have to do is look to the past. Did you know many of the 60's and 70's bodybuilders were training the entire body 2-3 times a week? 3 times a week is extreme for a normal person who has to work and earn a living, etc. So like me, you want something high impact, time friendly and results driven. The regime is spread over two weeks, training the body twice in the first week and once in the second, and repeat.

2 - Body Fat

There are a number of things you need to consider, to get the maximum out of your workouts. Your testosterone is utilized at its best when you have a lower body fat percentage. So this is the number one issue to deal with when beginning a new regime. A low body fat percentage gives you more utilization. This is also why the workouts are supersets. We are ramping up your intensity and effort to burn additional calories.

3 - Nutrition

Nutrition is considered the most important part of building muscle. If the nutrition is incorrect, then it doesn't matter how impeccable your training routines are, you will not progress. I'm sure you have an idea about nutrition, but I'm here to give your knowledge a little boost. You've heard of high protein, carbohydrates and healthy fats? But what are the most effective foods to eat to get those essential nutrients? This equals feeding your muscles exactly what they need and therefore means you will build muscle.

Last but not least is a high water intake. This cleans our systems, regulates body temperature and keeps the entire body hydrated. So with heavy exercise, 3 liters a day is an ideal figure to aim for. This isn't part of intermittent fasting, you can drink as much water as you like.

If you are over 50

Why exercising? Considering how easy it is to fast intermittently, you can easily squeeze in some exercise while you are at it. Especially in your fifties, you need to work to preserve your muscles. You have already lost plenty of muscle mass as you aged, so the importance of maintaining whatever muscle you have left is even more pronounced. Regular exercising will help you push your body beyond the limit of people your age, so you can do a little bit more than others, which is often the difference between you staying up or outside and staying in. Another added benefit of exercising is that it helps burn more fat, so there is no reason why you should consider skipping the exercise unless you have medical problems.

Just like intermittent fasting, the best exercise is the one that works for you. At your age, sticking to lightweight exercise or aerobic exercise is ideal because you will not put a lot of stress on your body. Jogging, cycling, or swimming are perfect.

A training session should consist of a warm-up, the actual training, and the cooldown phase. During the warm-up phase, you need to activate your muscles by moving your arms or legs at a gentle pace to prepare them for more vigorous movements later. It should last between 10 to 15 minutes. The bulk of your training should last for 30 minutes. The cooldown phase should last between 10 to 15 minutes, during which you need to stretch your muscles to let them relax.

PART III

NEW LIFE FOREVER

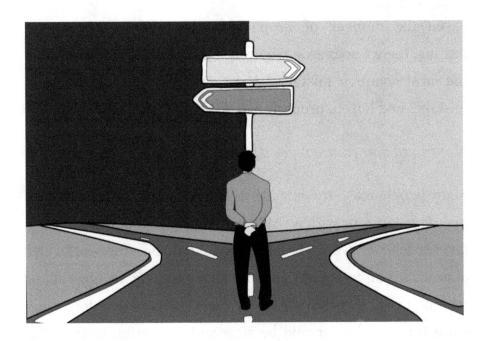

Routine

Your body will eventually get used to your intermittent fasting method. Once it gets used to it, you will eventually stop progressing in losing weight. This is easily solved by switching to the other intermittent fasting methods. It is important that you keep your body guessing and prevent it from getting used to a routine.

Mistakes to avoid

Given the number of people who have tried Intermittent Fasting, there's no reason why you should have to suffer through the most common mistakes! Here are 4 of the most common mistakes and how to properly avoid them.

Not breaking fast correctly!

Many people make the mistake of breaking fast with something high in calories or with a really big serving or a portion of their favorite food. However, breaking fast should be a thoughtful and almost meditative event that's not about gorging, feeling full, or rushing to eat. Breaking fast, especially if it's been a long time since you've eaten, should be slow and respectful, to both the food and to your body. Don't cram in the calories or eat a lot right away! Your body doesn't want **or need** that type of treatment. Start with a small something or eat slowly through a big portion, so that your body can adjust without cramps or aches and pains. Be thoughtful and don't rush to avoid this common mistake.

Wasting your eating window!

Some people turn to Intermittent Fasting because their days are hectic already and it makes sense not to eat all the time. Sometimes, people choose small eating windows, particularly because they don't normally eat a lot each day, to begin with. For people who make these sorts of choices especially, please be careful not to waste valuable eating time! It might seem like you can work forever and push off eating until later and later and later, but sometimes, you could push it off until the eating window is totally gone, and your body certainly won't thank you for that. Be mindful of your timing and of when you're supposed to eat. Respect that allotment of time for what it can give to your body: health, nourishment, and energy.

Trying too much at once!

Some people try to fast while dieting and while seriously exercising, and they wonder why they have no energy left! People who **want** to live high-intensity lifestyles like this are best suited toward plans like 5:2 (making sure not to exercise on those two fast days!). But even so, these individuals shouldn't put their bodies through **too much** stress with the addition of Intermittent Fasting. If you are attempting to do all three (diet, fast, and exercise), and you notice your energy level dropping, your mood swinging, or your belly burning, it might be time to cut back on one of those elements. Do a little less exercise! Eat a little more when you can! Try to add in some more calories! IF isn't about starvation, and it should never lead to that when done correctly and with healthy intentions. Remember that as you proceed with your journey.

Giving up too soon!

It's often the case that people give up on IF before the first week is over. They're frustrated by these feelings of hunger, and they feel convinced they'll never see results. Don't be duped into this way of thinking! Remember the power of your will. Be stubborn! Push through that first week and look forward to seeing results. They sometimes aren't as immediate as you'd hope, but that doesn't mean they're not coming! Even if you can tell the method you chose isn't working, try to last out the first week before troubleshooting and choosing a different one. For people who aren't convinced even after switching methods, try to go a whole two weeks before giving up entirely. You never know—it could be that last day in two weeks that your body starts to show results! Keep a focused mindset and a clear eye on your goals. Push through any hardship and be stubborn with your hopes and actions! Success will come in time.

Ignoring previous eating issues or disorders

There is nothing more harmful than the possible consequences if one chose to do an intermittent fast despite a history with eating disorders. Consult your doctor first before doing intermittent fasting. Also, seek alternative weight loss strategies that you can do.

Getting into it too fast

If this is your first weight loss plan, it is best to slowly get into intermittent fasting. Any diet or eating regimen will cause stress to your mind. If you are used to eating every two to four hours, you would not have a good experience jumping into a 16-hour fast immediately.

It is best to start with a shorter fasting period. You can start by reducing your number of meals. You can set a maximum number of meals for the day and set a schedule for it that you would follow. Once you get used to it, you can start by delaying your breakfast for a two to four hours in the morning. You can then adjust it until you reach the desired number of hours for your fasting period.

Not taking nutritional supplements

Regardless of how much food and variety is in your meals, it is difficult to acquire the full spectrum of vitamins and minerals for your body. You would need to take nutritional supplements if you want to your body to get the best nourishment. You can get what you would generally need from a daily multivitamin, a fish oil supplement (or similar omega-3 supplements), calcium supplement, and vitamin D supplement.

Eating too much carbohydrates and/or protein

Eating too many carbohydrates or protein than you need will cause your body to store excess energy into body fat. If you are not losing fat with intermittent fasting, you are probably making this mistake.

Generally, your total calorie intake for a day should consist of 45 to 65 percent of carbohydrates while 25 to 35 percent of protein. If you are aiming for fat loss, your carbohydrate intake should be lower while your protein consumption should increase.

Too much fat in the diet

If you eat too much fat, your body will prioritize burning the fat from your diet for energy. Again, you will find it difficult to lose weight and body fat if this is the case. To avoid this, keep your dietary fat intake to 20 to 35 percent of your total daily calories.

Eating too much calories

The intermittent fasting will put you on a calorie deficit. This is how you will lose fat. If you eat too much calories, you will find it difficult to lose fat and even experience weight gain.

To avoid eating too much, do not eat foods that will increase your appetite like keto bombs and salty food. You can also add more fiber and lean protein in your diet since it will help you feel more full.

Also, if you find yourself looking forward to breaking your fast, you might not be ready for your fasting schedule. Start with a shorter fasting period and gradually build it up.

Not enough calories

You do not need to restrict your calories in intermittent fasting. Your body will do it for you by feeling satiated after a meal. Restricting calories in intermittent fasting will just result in having too little calories available for your needs. Your body will respond by slowing down its metabolism, which will lead to weight gain.

The solution to this is to eat a meal with an amount close to how much you normally eat from a single meal without intermittent fasting.

Feeling too hungry

If you feel abnormally hungry in the middle or at the end of your fast, your fasting method is not suitable for your body's current state. This is usually the case for individuals who are not yet keto-adapted. This often results to overeating or eating anything even if its low quality calories.

To avoid this, start with a 10 or 12-hour fasting period and increase the time once you can go through it without being bothered by hunger.

Lack of exercise

Exercise provides a lot of benefits for your health. Not doing it due to intermittent fasting is the contrary to your pursuit of a healthier life. You have to figure out on how you can do it with intermittent fasting and just do it.

Walking and resistance training are the best forms of exercise with intermittent fasting. Walking would not increase your stress levels while resistance training will increase your growth hormone production.

Stressful lifestyle

High emotional and physical stress will increase cortisol levels. If you combine this with intermittent fasting, you will like lose lean muscle mass, and gain weight from fat. This elevated stress is often a combination of poor sleep, poor stress management, and a busy lifestyle. If you cannot fix these causes for your increased stress, it might be best to handle these issues first before doing intermittent fasting.

Drinking Bulletproof coffee

Some would suggest that drinking Bulletproof coffee would not break your fast, but this belief is completely wrong. Bulletproof coffee contains butter and MCT oil. Both of these contain calories.

Drinking Bulletproof coffee will not break your fast since it does not change your blood sugar levels, but it will stop you from losing weight. Since you introduced butter and MCT oil into your body as sources of fat, the body will stop using your body fat to make ketone bodies for energy.

Drink more water

Water keeps you hydrated and makes you feel fuller when you are on your fast. Being in a fasted state also acts as a diuretic, which means that your body will naturally expel water at a faster rate than you are used to. For best results, it's recommended that you drink a gallon of water.

CHAPTER 14: HOW TO COMBINE INTERMITTENT FASTING WITH JOB & FAMILY

Support of the family

Things are always easier with support. Some of us like to think that we're eagles, living solo among all the turkeys. We want to be free without anyone there to back us up. We don't need them! But this isn't ideal, especially when things are difficult. Sometimes, it's better to be surrounded by turkeys who care about you and will support you. Sometimes it's better to be the turkey because you know you're lovingly supported by your friends and family with you. What I'm trying to say here is that when you struggle with intermittent fasting, having the support of your friends can really make a difference in your success or failure.

If you have some friends who are very supportive of you, make sure they know when you're struggling with your fasting goals. They can probably give you a good shoulder to cry on and may even give you some tips for how to make things easier. If you're very lucky, your friends may join your fast with you. This way, you can keep each other accountable. If they don't want to fast, that's okay too, so long as they're supportive of you following your health goals.

If you're truly an eagle, alone in the world, then seek support from online communities. There are a lot of blogs and forums out there, dedicated to intermittent fasting. Join some of them and talk to others who are struggling. Some great forums to join include the Reddit forum on intermittent fasting. There, they post pictures of success, questions about speed bumps, and even give each other motivation. Get involved and you'll have some support too.

How to plan Intermittent Fasting with working hours

Here are the guides that may help in doing intermittent fasting:

Start with a shorter, daily intermittent fast

This is the easier way to start fasting. Limit food intake to about 8 hours each day. Recommended times are between 12 noon to 8 pm.

Make lunch as the day's first meal. Then after dinner (around 8pm), stop taking food. This is easy because the first 8 hours of fast is spent sleeping. Upon waking up, skip breakfast. If caffeine is needed to start the day, go ahead and drink coffee. It does not have to be a decaf, or black, or no sugar. Whatever type of caffeine source needed, go ahead and take it. There is no need to stress about it. All day, one can eat and drink anything. There is no need to think about zero-calorie drinks or non-fat milk or any of that other stuff. Eat a hearty dinner. Then go on a fast again from bedtime until lunchtime the next day.

Shorter daily fast and feeding windows have more consistent eating schedules. This will not overwhelm the body when adapting to the changes in eating pattern. It is easier to focus on making healthy food choices during the feeding window. For those with metabolic or blood sugar concerns, short daily fast/feeding is less stressful.

Give the body some time to adjust

At first, it will be a bit difficult to limit the food consumption to certain periods a day. This is only temporary, as the body shifts to fat burning for fuel. Keeping busy will help keep the mind from hunger and thoughts of food. The more difficult part is controlling the food portions during the eating periods. Eat food slowly to avoid overeating. Curb cravings for high energy snacks like sweets by opting for healthier snacks like fruits. Give the body time to recognize and adapt to this new food intake pattern. This may only take a few days.

Go for longer intermittent fasting periods

As the body learns to rely on fat burning as an energy source, other than fast sources like carbohydrates, try to lengthen the fast periods. From a 16-hour fast, gradually lengthen it to 24 hours. Do it twice a week. Eat normally for 5 days, and then schedule 2 days a week for 24-hour fast periods. The 2 days of fasting should not be consecutive. Space it over the entire week.

Longer intermittent fasting once or twice a week, allows a person to have better calorie intake on eating days. Remember that intermittent fasting is not a crash diet where food intake is severely restricted. On fast days, meals can be kept simple. Consume only about a quarter (or about 600 calories) on these days. Longer fasting periods also allows for deeper cellular cleansing or detoxification.

Watch out for overeating after fasting days. This is common, as the body tries to compensate for the longer periods of low food intake. Also, make conscious healthier food choices on eating days. There is a tendency to put less focus on the type of food consumed during "normal" days. Junk foods and processed foods should still be avoided. Also, refrain from food that contains bad types of fats.

Get some exercise

Fat burning is maximized when exercising during the fast periods. There is better metabolic adaptation. It improves muscle protein synthesis, hence, better lean muscle build up.

Meals taken after fasted training are quickly metabolized as the body recovers, both from the fasted state and from the rigors of exercise. However, allow the body to adjust first to intermittent fasting. Then, gradually increase the intensity of exercise during the fasting days.

keto & IF

What is Keto diet

The new hype low carbohydrate, adequate-protein, and high-fat diet is keto diet. The idea of the keto diet is to restrict carbohydrate intake, so the body could burn fat instead of glucose. The fat burning choice is making food more prevalent among people who want to lose weight. The low carb diet, not only helps you lose weight, but also improves your health. The ketogenic diet may even have benefits against Epilepsy, Cancer, Alzheimer's disease, and Diabetes.

Unlike any other diet, Keto has its unique lifestyle requirements. Keto Diet is different and a little bit complicated.

To get your body into a ketogenic state, you should eat a high-fat diet and low protein with NO carbs or scarcely any. The proportion ought to be around 80% fats and 20% protein. It will be the rule for the initial two days.

Basics and rules for Keto Diet

A typical breakdown of a keto diet would be Fat: 70%, Carbs: 5%, and Protein: 25%.

Your daily net carbs intake should be 20-30 gram to stay in Ketosis.

Limit your fruit consumption to avocados, berries, and coconut.

Drink more water. You need to drink 2-3 litres of water daily.

Say no to carb dressings, spreads, sweeteners, or high carb nuts.

Make sure you are eating no carbs at all, and also, keep track of your meal intake.

Eat fatty breakfast and eat one fat in each meal.

Stock your pantry with healthy foods, i.e., meat, eggs, starchy vegetables, avocados, saturated fats, like, coconut oil, ghee, olive oil, sesame oil, flaxseed oil.

Eat raw dairy, but if you are allergic, avoid it.

Soak and dehydrate nuts before you eat them.

Drink Bone Broth every day.

Increase your electrolytes (sodium, magnesium, and potassium) intake to keep yourself safe from Keto flu.

Plan and track your diet carefully.

Differences and similarities with Intermittent Fasting

Do you know what the best thing about intermittent fasting is? Weight loss and better health are undoubtedly good reasons; however, the answer is autophagy. Do you know what autophagy is? Read on to learn more about autophagy and how intermittent fasting helps.

There are different reasons why people opt for intermittent fasting, and the reasons can range from weight loss to convenience. Restricting yourself to an eating window of just a couple of hours daily puts your body into a state of calorie deficit, but using intermittent fasting to lose weight is merely a partial benefit.

Juice cleanses and detox diets don't work. They are merely fad diets, and like all fads, they will fade away. There is nothing wrong with having a kale smoothie to flush the toxins out of your system; however, there is a better way to get rid of toxins. Our bodies can cleanse themselves, and it is via a process that you can fully control. All you need to do is trigger the self-cannibalism metabolism of your body. It might sound slightly scary, but it is quite natural and perfect for your overall health. Does that seem dubious? It isn't, and you can train your body to eat itself. It is known as autophagy, and it helps to cleanse your body. Apart from all the toxins in the body, there are plenty of dead and diseased cells as well.

In autophagy, your body gobbles up these cells and helps to make new ones in their place. You have to send your car for servicing from time to time, even if it functions well. You have to replace the oil in your car, and certain new parts have to be installed. In the same manner, your body needs to be serviced from time to time to make it more efficient. The faulty parts would need to be removed, and new ones put in their place. Well, autophagy does this for you.

Autophagocytosis is the technical term for autophagy. Autophagy might sound slightly scary, but it is an entirely natural process. It is a body mechanism that helps to disassemble our cells and get rid of all their components that are dysfunctional. It essentially means that your body is in a recycle mode and gets rid of all the waste that's accumulated within. Autophagy places your body in a catabolic state wherein it starts to break down its tissue instead of an anabolic state where it builds tissue.

There are plenty of benefits that autophagy offers. It helps to reduce inflammation in the body and strengthens your immune system. Autophagy also slows down the process of aging and suppresses the growth of cancerous cells and tumors. It also kills any infectious particles and toxins present in the body. The lack of autophagy leads to weight gain, laziness, impairment of the brain and high levels of cholesterol.

So, how does autophagy work? When your body triggers autophagy, the cells present in your body hunt for all the dead or malfunctioning cells and destroys them. Destroy might not be the right word; the healthy cells devour the unhealthy cells. It involves the creation of a double membrane around a cell that's going to be eaten, and it is known as an autophagosome. The diseased cell or the toxic protein is dissolved by the autophagosome, and it produces energy. How does your body regulate autophagy? The main triggers of autophagy are two types of protein enzymes known as mTOR and AMPK. mTOR is responsible for the growth of cells and the synthesis of proteins as well as anabolism. It helps to activate the insulin receptors in the body and helps the body create new tissue. AMPK activates a protein kinase that helps to balance energy levels when energy levels in the body are depleted.

How does intermittent fasting support autophagy? Intermittent fasting helps to trigger autophagy due to caloric deficiency. The reduction in the calorie intake helps the healthy cells to get rid of unnecessary proteins, and break these down to release amino acids that provide energy. Intermittent fasting helps to improve your overall health, and prolongs your lifespan as well. Autophagy is the main reason for the benefits that intermittent fasting provides. Autophagy kicks in due to calorie restriction. You might wonder if a diet that prescribes small meals with little calorie intake might have similar benefits; however, it doesn't work like that. If you continuously provide your body with nutrition, it cannot enter autophagy. Two conditions are essential to autophagy. The first condition is the reduction of calorie intake and the second condition is a period of fast. When you fast, your body reaches for its reserves to provide energy. If you continuously supply it fuel, it doesn't have to process any fats or process any additional proteins. Your body is better off without any calories while you fast, instead of breaking the fast with a couple of calories and efficiently stopping autophagy. It is a good idea to follow the protocols of intermittent fasting, if not daily, then at least a couple of times a week.

Imagine if you have three square meals daily. You stop eating at 8 p.m., and you fast throughout the night. The first morsel of food you consume will be at 8 a.m. the following day. There is a gap of 12 hours between your meals; however, your body needs anywhere between 6 to 8 hours to fully digest the food you eat before it can shift into a fasted state. In practice, your fast doesn't start until the middle of the night, and you fast for only 6 hours. That isn't much time for your body to start autophagy. When your body is in a fed state, autophagy is low because of insulin and mTOR. Only when the fuel in your body decreases, does autophagy start. There is no fixed time for when autophagy starts. It varies according to the tissues in the body. As a rule of thumb, autophagy starts only when your insulin and mTOR levels are low. It doesn't happen when your body glucose levels are high. Your body needs to be in a state of mild ketosis with low levels of liver glycogen for this process to start. It can take anywhere between 12 to 16 hours for autophagy to set in; however, the process amps up after a couple of days of fasting.

However, it doesn't mean that you must starve yourself and stop eating altogether. If you do this, then you run the risk of starving your body, and it will negatively affect all the other activities you perform. Fasting doesn't lead to the loss of muscle, due to an increase in growth hormones and the production of ketones in the body. Autophagy is essential to maintain muscle mass.

Your body can enter into autophagy if you do the following.

Try to fast for a period of 14 to 16 hours daily to put your body in a fasted state. It will allow the depletion of glycogen reserves in your body and keep your body in a state of mild ketosis all day long. You must keep your insulin levels low in the blood. If you keep eating carbs or protein, then you will suppress autophagy; however, if you consume more fats, then you will contain the insulin response in your body and help to prolong the benefits of fasting. It might briefly stop autophagy, but it does put your body in ketosis. Ketosis helps to reduce inflammation and boosts the health of cells. Regardless of what you decide to do, don't binge on carbs. If you don't want to trigger the release of insulin and mTOR, then you must control your carb intake. Exercise also helps to stimulate autophagy in the body.

A little bit of self-destruction and stress are necessary to empower your body to function well. Self-destruction doesn't mean anything that puts you in mortal danger. It is a simple process that your body follows to cleanse and rid itself of additional proteins.

Researchers and nutrition specialists are stating in new articles and books the point that the future way of keeping weight off or losing weight is intermittent fasting, and these are being distributed every day including the smash hit books like 'Eat

Stop Eat' and 'The 8 Hour Diet'. Irregular fasting is likewise well known with supporters of the Paleo diet since our progenitors seem to have eaten along these lines for a great many years.

WHAT IS I.F.?

Irregular fasting is an eating regimen plan where you quit for a set timeframe during the day. This is generally between 16-20 consecutive hours. Within 4-8 hours

daily, you can eat.

When fasting, you can drink low calorie or without calorie sustenances. Think espresso, tea, water, and vegetables.

The additional time you go fast daily, the better results you get. You can do these regularly to your liking. Once more, your results are better, and are as regular as you fast.

CHAPTER 16: HOW TO COMBINE INTERMITTENT FASTING WITH KETO DIET

Benefits of Intermittent fasting with Ketosis

The ketogenic diet helps your body maintain a fat-burning state. It consists of low carbohydrate, moderate protein, and high fat proportions. This dietary composition causes similar benefits to intermittent fasting, since it uses the same mechanics of reducing insulin resistance, stimulating fat metabolism, and promoting autophagy in the body. Because of their similar effects, you might find yourself wondering if you can do both at the same time.

The short answer to this is YES. You can combine the keto diet and intermittent fasting. However, it will be difficult. Therefore, it is best that you have consistently done one of these two for a few months before combining it with the other. Here are the rules that you have to follow for a ketogenic diet:

Macronutrient proportions are at 75 percent fat, 20% protein, and 5% carbohydrates.

Macronutrient proportions are based on a person's daily caloric needs to maintain weight.

You are restricted from food and beverage containing sugar, simple carbohydrates, alcohol, citrus, and fructose.

Other forms of sugar are not allowed, such as maple syrup, honey, coconut sugar, and agave syrup.

Starchy vegetables, beans, legumes, grains, and grain products are not prohibited.

Unhealthy fats, like margarine and vegetable oils, should be avoided.

Processed and packaged foods are not allowed.

Food and drinks with sweeteners, preservatives, and artificial coloring in the ingredients should be avoided.

When combining a ketogenic diet with intermittent fasting, you have to make sure that you are getting enough calories and nutrients. You have to be sure that you are eating enough calories. Since you will be restricted from eating carbohydrates, you have to place an emphasis on your diet for nutrient-dense keto-approved food items. These include food high in healthy fat like avocado, high quality animal and plant source of protein, coconut oil, and leafy green vegetables.

Furthermore, you have to closely track the levels of your ketone bodies. You need to stay in ketosis without reaching the levels that indicate diabetic ketoacidosis (240 mg/dl). Because of this risk, you need to use glucose meters with a ketone measurement feature. Warning signs of diabetic ketoacidosis include vomiting for more than two hours, queasy feeling, stomachache, fruity breath, difficulty breathing, tiredness, dizziness, and confusion.

Lastly, you have to take a similar approach to how you started intermittent fasting. You have to take it slow. In this case, you will gradually decrease carbohydrates in your diet. This will help your body get used to having no access to carbohydrates and to being in an almost constant state of ketosis.

The same precautions from intermittent fasting apply in this combination with the keto diet. You have to observe how your body is doing. You have to make sure that you do not feel like you are not getting enough calories. You also have to ensure that you feel well doing it. Lastly, you have to adjust the diet and the fasting length if you ever find it necessary to do so.

Benefits of Keto Diet

Loss in weight

"There is anecdotal evidence that people lose weight through the keto diet," says Melinda R. Ring, MD, director of the Northwestern Medicine Osher Center for Integrative Medicine.

No low-fat food anymore

On paper, burning fats by eating more fats is tempting, which is why the keto diet has become so popular. The keto diet allows many people to eat the types of high-fat foods they enjoy, such as red meat, fatty fish, nuts, cheese, and butter, while still losing weight.

Health benefits for certain people

The keto diet helps to reduce seizures in pediatric patients with epilepsy. Endurance athletes and bodybuilders also use keto to lose fat in a short time. The keto diet is being studied to alleviate the symptoms in patients with progressive neurological conditions such as Parkinson's disease. Still, scientific research has not confirmed the benefit of these populations.

Type 2 diabetes

The carbohydrate limitation can have a direct effect on glucose concentration and reduce it over time. It can be a simple way to control your diabetes

But you should consult a registered dietitian before applying this strategy. Generally, a healthy diet and carbohydrate control can give the same results.

Cancer

There is a growing field of research for the keto diet. The Warburg effect has shown that tumor cells can break down glucose much faster (200x faster) than typical cells. The theory is that starving tumor cells from glucose can inhibit their growth and prevent cancer.

Keto is ideal for a predominantly sedentary lifestyle

Sedentary lifestyles are too common - a lifestyle often dictated by desk jobs and long hours. Even if you exercise for about 30 minutes in a day and the rest of the day are rather inactive, there are good reasons to keep carbohydrate intake low because you do not need muscle glycogen.

In addition, you can make the carbohydrates you have work more efficiently for you by scheduling your intake around your pre-workout and post-workout plan.

We can consider as benefits:

1) Accelerated fat burning

Avoiding sugar Carbohydrates is one of the most effective ways to lose much fat, and thus, excess body weight in a short time.

The reason is that low-carb diets in the first step remove excess water from your body, then lower your insulin levels, and ultimately reduce your hunger/appetite.

In the long run, ketosis transforms your body into a fat-burning machine that operates 24 hours a day, 7 days a week.

2) Stable and low blood sugar level

Millions of people all over the world suffer from diabetes or high insulin resistance. The best thing for these people is that the ketogenic diet can provide some benefits.

Avoiding carbohydrates can dramatically decrease your blood sugar levels, preventing fatigue or starvation.

3) Increased stamina

Even endurance athletes can boost their performance through ketosis. This is because energy production from ketones and fatty acids consumes less oxygen and is generally more efficient.

The FASTER study is one of the best-known and large-scale studies in this field. The researchers studied the effects of ketosis on the endurance of athletes - with amazing results.

In summary, the keto athletes differed by more powerful mitochondria, accelerated fat burning, less oxygen demand, and a slightly increased efficiency.

4) Better sleep quality

Sleep and especially deep sleep has been proven to be one of the most important processes in our body. Again, ketosis can work wonders!

This is because ketosis activates cell-internal "garbage collection" on the one hand, and on the other hand, leads to efficient energy production. Therefore, Ketarier often enables a better quality of sleep and a decrease in the need for sleep.

5) Improved brain functions

Another well-researched advantage of the ketogenic diet is the enhancement of brain functions such as memory, concentration, or focus.

Several human studies have confirmed the beneficial effects of ketosis on the memory of adults.

Besides, ketosis leads to an increase in the production of mitochondria in the human brain, which can increase the concentration of ATP in the brain, and especially in your hippocampus.

6) Higher metabolic rate and energy consumption

Basal metabolic rate is the amount of energy your body requires per day to keep the most important functions going in your body.

Some studies have linked low carb or ketogenic diet to higher basal metabolic rates. This means that weight can be lost faster in the long term to define the body or muscles.

7) Nutrient-rich diet

Foods that should be eaten in the ketogenic diet include fish, vegetables, high-quality meat, and other unrefined foods.

These foods are rich in minerals and required nutrients that contribute to the health and performance of your body.

8) Lower blood pressure

Just as exciting: hypertensive patients can benefit from a ketogenic diet.

It is confirmed that a low-carb diet and forms of the ketogenic diet can reduce some important risk factors of various heart diseases. This includes lower blood pressure.

9) Stronger mitochondria

Mitochondria are the cell power plants of our bodies. Without them, the energy would go out within a few minutes. Most of our health, performance, and immune system rely on the function of our mitochondria.

In general, one can conclude from their research that ketosis can measurably increase the performance and number of mitochondria in the body.

10) Slower aging process

One way to mitigate the aging of the body is to reduce oxidative stress. Interestingly, low insulin levels lead to less oxidative stress.

Avoiding sugar and other carbohydrates as part of a ketogenic diet will sustainably lower the blood sugar and insulin levels in the body, which in turn will measurably and noticeably slow down your aging process.

11) Faster and stronger satiety

Many diets cause one thing above all else: a constant feeling of hunger. The keto diet is different here - because it can be proven to lead to a stronger feeling of satiety, which also occurs even faster.

Several studies show that carbohydrate wasting and consumption of more fat and protein results in less hunger and a lower calorie count every year.

This will allow you to burn fat in less time - without the unpleasant feeling of constant and ubiquitous hunger!

12) Fasting becomes much easier

Everyone knows the feeling when we give up our lunch or forgot about dinner because of hard work.

As part of a normal diet, most people find it hard to forego any food for 12 hours even though fasting can have incredible health benefits. It's different in ketosis: it's no longer a problem if you do not eat for 12, 16, or even 24 hours. As a result, prolonged or intermittent fasting (16-hour daily fasting) will be much easier.

13) Better mood & mood

There are many effects of the ketogenic diet on people with autism.

Among other things, this effect is due to the increased formation of GABA and serotonin in the course of ketosis. The distribution of these happy hormones, in turn, means that Ketarier often reports an improved mood.

Another convincing reason to forego sugar and simple carbohydrates in the future!

14) Faster weight loss

It has been scientifically proven that low carb and high-fat diets are the most efficient way to lose plenty of weight and fat in a short period of time.

On the one hand, this is because so much water (which is bound to carbohydrates and glycogen) is excreted.

Second, you turn your body into an efficient fat-burning machine. In this way, you will burn fat faster and more effectively over the long term and lose weight.

15) Higher HDL cholesterol

HDL cholesterol (high-density lipoprotein) is also often referred to as the good cholesterol. The higher the amount of HDL, relative to the "bad" LDL, the lower the risk of heart disease.

Through the high consumption of healthy fatty acids in the course of the ketogenic diet, you can raise the amount of "good" HDL cholesterol and thus prevent heart disease.

16) Increased libido

Ketosis can significantly increase the quality of life of men through increased testosterone levels and more libidos.

This effect gets stronger the more high-quality fats (MCT, coconut fat, etc.) you eat like a man in ketosis.

17) Lower insulin levels

Low-carb diets and ketogenic nutrition are particularly beneficial to people with diabetes and high insulin resistance - these conditions affect several million people worldwide.

Studies have shown that people suffering from diabetes can reduce their insulin levels by up to 50 percent with a low / no-carb diet.

18) Faster getting up in the morning

Because of the improved sleep quality that we wrote about earlier in the article, many Ketarians report more energy and willpower to get them out of bed in the morning.

19) Improved LDL cholesterol level

People with too high an LDL level are more likely to have a heart attack during their lifetime.

In ketosis, the size of LDL particles rises, while the absolute number of particles mitigates. As the LDL particles become larger, the lower the risk of myocardial infarction.

Therefore, by avoiding sugar and carbohydrates, you can reduce the risk of a heart attack!

20) Reduces symptoms of allergies

In addition, ketosis balances and soothes the human immune system. Since an allergy is nothing but an overreaction of the immune system, ketosis can reduce the symptoms of allergies.

21) Ketose has an anticatabolic effect

Athletes especially, are afraid to lose hard-earned muscle mass in ketosis

Ketones have an anticatabolic effect in your body. This means giving signal to your body that it should not reduce muscle but fat.

Benefits of Intermittent Diet

1.Weight Loss

The vast majority of people who try intermittent fasting are using it to help them lose weight.

This works in two ways; firstly by reducing the number of overall calories being consumed, and secondly by improving hormone function that promotes weight loss.

This is due to the lowering of insulin levels along with the increase of norepinephrine, which is a growth hormone. This combination increases the metabolic rate and causes body fat to be broken down and used for energy.

The benefit of this double action is that weight loss is being promoted from two sides of the equation. The calories you are using are being increased, and the calories you are consuming are being reduced.

Most individuals see weight loss of between 3% and 8% over a three to twenty-four week period. If you look at it from another perspective and measure your waist circumference to gauge the amount of harmful belly fat lost, it can range between 4% and 7% in the same period.

2. Reduces Insulin Resistance and Risk of Type 2 Diabetes

The instance of type 2 diabetes has shown a dramatic rise in recent years. This is thought to be mostly due to poor diet and the consumption of foods that cause insulin levels to become raised over long periods, thereby causing firstly, insulin resistance, and eventually resulting in type 2 diabetes.

Our body's primary energy source is glucose, which we get from the food we eat. In recent times, the amount of glucose-producing foods we consume has increased dramatically.

High carbohydrate processed foods are one of the biggest causes, and they include breakfast cereals, white bread, white pasta, white rice and products made with refined wheat flour such as cakes, cookies, and pastries. These foods are rapidly broken down into glucose in the body and the sheer volume that floods the system causes a big problem. Having too much glucose in the bloodstream is bad news, and the body wants to use it up as fast as possible. To achieve this Insulin is released into the body; it helps it use up the glucose for energy, as well as taking it to your liver, muscles and (if there is too much, which there usually is) your fat cells.

To give you the basic idea, insulin works by rushing around your body telling all the cells "Hey guys, look, there's lots of glucose here for you to use as energy!" At first, the cells respond and take in the glucose, but quickly they become full and don't want any more, so they start ignoring the message that the insulin is giving them. The body's reaction to this is to release more insulin to try to convince the cells to take the glucose. The insulin levels are raised higher and higher and over a period of time, you become insulin resistant. Eventually, this can lead to type 2 diabetes.

Intermittent fasting can reverse insulin resistance and reduce blood sugar levels, thereby avoiding type 2 diabetes and kidney damage.

3. Cells, Genes, and Hormones

Fasting causes your body to initiate a cellular repair process and changes hormone levels that allow body fat to be used as energy more easily.

This is what happens during fasting:

Insulin. The level of insulin in the blood drops significantly, allowing fat to be more easily used for energy.

Human Growth Hormone. The amount of human growth hormone circulating in the blood increases to up to 5 times the normal levels. This increase allows fat to be used as an energy source and muscle mass to be *increased*.

Cellular Repair. The cells of the body become more active, repairing themselves and eliminating waste materials.

Gene Expression. Due to the beneficial effects fasting has on gene expression and the function of hormones and cells, it is anticipated that intermittent fasting practices may not only protect against diseases but actually increase longevity.

4. Inflammation and Oxidative Stress

Many chronic diseases, as well as aging, can be promoted by oxidative stress. This is when free radicals, which are unstable molecules, interact with other important molecules such as proteins and even DNA, thus damaging them.

When combined with a diet that is high in antioxidant-rich foods, intermittent fasting may help your body becomes more resistant to oxidative stress.

Inflammation, which is a fundamental cause of many common diseases, can also be reduced by intermittent fasting. A study published in the online issue 16 of Nature Medicine, describes how β-hydroxybutyrate inhibits a complex set of proteins known as inflammasome, particularly NLRP3. The inflammasome is responsible for driving inflammatory response in disorders such as type 2 diabetes, Alzheimer's disease, autoimmune diseases, atherosclerosis, and other autoinflammatory disorders.

5. Heart Health

The biggest killer in the world is currently heart disease. Intermittent fasting can improve many of the risk factors associated with heart disease, including LDL cholesterol levels, blood pressure, triglycerides, inflammation, and blood sugar levels. This provides a useful way to help prevent the disease on the long term. This is particularly useful for people who have a family history of heart disease.

Unfortunately, because intermittent fasting is of no interest to the pharmaceutical industry (because they can't make money from it), very little study has been done on humans to ascertain the full effects that intermittent fasting can provide. In order to really understand the full potential, a lot more human trials need to be done.

6. Cellular Repair

Cellular repair, known as autophagy, is stimulated by fasting. Autophagy is when all the dysfunctional and broken proteins that have accumulated within the cells over time are broken down and eliminated.

Autophagy can help protect the body against diseases such as Alzheimer's and cancer.

7. Cancer

Another disease that seems to have become more prevalent in recent times is cancer.

Cancer is the uncontrolled growth of cells, as the cells auto-destruct mechanism stops functioning and the cells continue to grow unhindered.

It is thought that when the body is in a fasting state that cancer cells cannot simply "wait out" the fast in the same way as normal cells do. Because they are permanently stuck in "on" mode, they cannot find the nutrients they need to sustain them during a fast. The healthy cells are unaffected, as they simply hibernate during the fast, which cancer cells cannot do.

Fasting is also useful for cancer prevention, as it reduces insulin resistance that is linked to several cancers. It also causes autophagy, where the cells clean out all the garbage, making them healthier.

As with heart disease, insufficient studies have been conducted to show the full potential of intermittent fasting in humans. We are now reliant on individual health associations to initiate the types of studies that are required to further prove the evidence gained to date.

8. Brain Health

The metabolic boost that intermittent fasting provides isn't only good for the body, it is good for the brain as well.

Oxidative stress, inflammation, blood sugar levels and insulin resistance, all have negative effects on brain health. Intermittent fasting has been shown to generate new nerve cells that benefit brain function.

A brain hormone, brain-derived neurotrophic factor (BDNF) is increased with intermittent fasting. Deficiency in this hormone has been linked to depression and other mental health problems.

As intermittent fasting can also help to lower blood pressure to normal levels, it is helpful in the prevention of strokes and heart attack.

9. Alzheimer's Disease

Alzheimer's is the most common neurodegenerative disease and it is incurable. Prevention is, therefore, most definitely the best approach.

Patients with Alzheimer's can benefit and show significant improvements when following short daily fasts.

Because fasting stimulates cell cleansing, it is believed that it can help to prevent the occurrence of disease and maintain brain health.

Other neurological diseases such as Parkinson's and Huntington's may also be prevented or improved with intermittent fasting.

As with most other diseases, more scientific research on humans is required to show the full potential intermittent fasting could have.

10. Longevity.

Most of us want to live a long and healthy life, and intermittent fasting could be one of the keys to helping you achieve this.

Fasting has been shown to extend the lifespan of rats in the same way as continuous calorie restriction increases lifespan. It was shown in one study published in the Journal of Nutrition, Volume 31, Issue 3, 1 March 1946, Pages 363–375, that rats fasted every other day lived 83% longer than rats that did not fast.

Although more research is necessary on human subjects, intermittent fasting has shown to be greatly popular amongst the anti-aging crowd.

Due to the positive effects on health, it isn't difficult to understand how intermittent fasting can help with an increased lifespan.

CONCLUSION

I hope this book helped you understand the basics of occasional fasting, and the benefits that this diet will bring into your life. By practicing occasional fasting while you are fit, and without having to adhere to strict diets that can be harmful to your health, you will succeed in reducing weight and be in the best form of your life.

Understanding the principles of occasional fasting, will not only help to reduce your weight, but it will also contribute to the strengthening of your mental health by training your brain to be durable and to resist food during moments that are meant for fasting. This way you will become a stronger person. However, the psyche is not the only thing that will be strengthened. Who does not want strong and well-shaped muscles? Well, occasional fasting will help in creating this. You must be wondering how something that deprives you of food can help you build muscle, when you know that building muscle requires more calorie intake. Well, this is not the case. Basically, intermittent fasting will teach you to appreciate food and to refer to a healthy diet that will become part of your everyday life. With the right combination of fat, carbohydrates, protein, fresh fruits and vegetables, you will be able to create meals that the body needs on the days you are not fasting.

The next step is to list all the various methods of intermittent fasting once more, to help you choose the one that will best suit your lifestyle and daily responsibilities, as well as gradually starting to change your life and taking care of your health forever. Of course, do not be alarmed if you are suddenly unable to endure the whole fasting period. Allow your body some time to get used to this way of eating, and over time you will be able to lengthen the time for fasting. Combine some simple exercises to increase the burning of fat from your body, or prepare your own exercise plan that will fit your fitness level. Nevertheless, try not to forget the recommendations given in the book, on the combination of the intensity of exercise during the days when you are fasting and the days when you are not fasting.

It is important to plan the exercise days very well. If you practice high-intensity workouts on the fasting day, you will feel exhausted, and your muscles will be under a lot of stress, which is not good when you are trying to shape and enhance. Also, to get those well-established and toned muscles, drink plenty of water (at least eight glasses, but really this is the minimum amount we need) and remember to combine protein, carbohydrates, and fat before and after training, to help your muscles grow. Take the recommendations of gradual entry into the process of fasting, and become one step closer to changing your whole life and becoming happier and satisfied with your visual appearance and health.

CPSIA information can be obtained
at www.ICGtesting.com
Printed in the USA
BVHW061805230321
603262BV00006B/518